FOREVER VITAL: The Timeless Guide to Thriving Through the Ages"

By

NEVILLE LAWSON

TABLE OF CONTENTS

Introduction

In the wide fabric of human experience, one enduring longing—the desire to live a fuller and longer life—has persisted across time. From the earliest civilizations to the highly modern society we live in today, humanity has always sought to push the boundaries of what is mortal. We have always desired to flourish despite the limitations imposed by time and the environment.

Welcome to"**Forever Vital:** The Timeless Guide to Thriving Through the Ages" Humanity has made enormous strides toward living longer, better, and happier lives, which are examined in this book. It delves into the enthralling past, forward-thinking discoveries, and bright future of health and science that promise to transform our conceptions of what it means to live a long life in the twenty-first century and beyond.

You will embark on an intriguing trip in the pages that follow that reveals the lasting appeal of long life for humans as well as the amazing developments that have spurred our unceasing hunt for it. We will look at the pioneers and visionaries who have pushed the boundaries of human existence, from the ancient alchemists seeking the elixir of life to the cutting-edge scientists of the present employing genetics and artificial intelligence to extend human life.

But this book isn't just a tour through the past. It acts as a road map for the day when science and medicine join forces to dramatically transform how we age. We'll look at the most recent advances in personalized medicine, regenerative medicine, and artificial intelligence, as well as the incredible potential of technologies like nanomedicine, gene editing, and nanotechnology to change the very essence of life itself.

In addition to being a book, "**FOREVER VITAL**" is a call to action.It makes us rethink our preconceived notions about aging and what it means to get older. In order to inspire us to recognize the entire range of human potential at every stage of life, we will challenge the cultural narratives that frequently limit how we view aging.

Prepare to be inspired, educated, and empowered as you explore the past, present, and future of aging and medicine. In order to ignite your desire to live above and beyond expectations, we want to create in you a spark—an ember of optimism that challenges conventional thinking about aging.

It is now vital to envision a society in which everyone can live longer, healthier, and more satisfying lives and in which growing older will only be a threshold to new opportunities and experiences rather than a fixed point. The book **"FOREVER VITAL"** encourages you to join us on this amazing adventure and explore the endless options that will open up as we reshape medicine and rethink the idea of healthy living for a longer and more satisfying life.

Chapter 1

Characterizing Life span and Its Significance

The nature of having a long life expectancy or presence is alluded to as life span. In spite of the fact that much of the time is about human existence, it can likewise be utilized to depict the life expectancy of a few different organic entities, ideas, associations, and, surprisingly, actual items. The idea of life span is intricate and incorporates a few aspects, including:

1. Human Lifespan: The protracting of human existence, anticipation and general wellbeing are the primary subjects of this angle. While it involves stretching an individual's life expectancy, it likewise focuses on the personal satisfaction over those extra years. A significant goal of medication, general wellbeing, and biomedical examination is broadening solid life expectancies.

2. Species Lifespan: This figure considers an animal groups' life span during development. Hereditary assortment, adaptability, and the ability to persevere through moving ecological circumstances are undeniably connected with species life span.

3. Hierarchical Life span: In the business world, an association's capacity to keep working and flourishing for quite a while is alluded to as its hierarchical life span. Procedures including imagination, transformation, and effective administration are habitually important to make long haul progress.

4. Philosophical and Social Life span: Social traditions, customs, and conviction designs can continue for some ages. In this sense, life span alludes to the support and dispersal of social heritage, values, and ideas.

Contingent upon the circumstance, the pertinence of life span could change, in spite of the fact that there are a few different ways it is huge:

1. Wellbeing and Prosperity: Expanding human lifespan is fundamental for increasing the expectation of living. The weight of constant sicknesses and handicaps in later life is reduced since it empowers individuals to live longer, better, and more useful lives.

2. Financial Effect: Carrying on with a long life can make critical financial impacts. Developing maturing populaces can come down on benefits plans and medical care frameworks, yet they can likewise open up new business sectors for organizations in the medical care, drug, and senior administrations areas.

3. The safeguarding of biodiversity and biological equilibrium relies upon the lifetime of species. The lifetime of an animal variety is impacted by endeavors to shield undermined

species and keep up with regular natural surroundings.

4. Sustainability: Life span and maintainability standards remain forever inseparable. The drawn out practicality of normal environments, undertakings, and networks is the objective of supportable practices and asset the executives.

5. Social Legacy: Social and philosophical life span is supported by the protection of social traditions, dialects, and verifiable data. Social orders can hold a sensation of progression and personality while likewise gaining from before.

6. Development and Progress: Versatility and advancement are habitually fundamental for life span. Long haul achievement and progression are bound to come to associations and civilizations that can change with the times and embrace new innovation.

Life span incorporates a large number of settings and is significant for some reasons, including cultural headway, monetary security, biodiversity insurance, maintainability, and individual and individual prosperity. Science, medical services, strategy, and endeavors to save social practices all assume significant parts in accomplishing life span.

A. The issue of life span in the public eye at large

Because of a few interrelated conditions, stretching out human existence has become a significant social worry on a worldwide scale. Think about the accompanying significant variables:

1. Maturing Populace: With a maturing populace, numerous countries are going through an immense segment disturbance. Lower rates of birth and longer futures are the fundamental variables driving this pattern. Longer life expectancies are an indication of further developed medical services and everyday environments, except they likewise bring new issues concerning medical services consumptions, benefits plans, and older consideration.

2. Expenses of Medical care: As individuals live longer, they frequently need more medical care administrations, especially as they age and the pervasiveness of constant illnesses rises. Worries about the maintainability of medical services spending are raised because of the huge monetary strain this puts on medical services frameworks and people.

3. Financial Ramifications: A maturing populace might influence efficiency and monetary development. A more modest workforce might bring about work deficiencies, less development, and higher reliance proportions (the extent of old wards to working-age individuals), which could come down on friendly wellbeing nets.

4. Social Government assistance Frameworks: Legislatures all over the planet are fighting to keep up with the reasonability of social government assistance frameworks, for example, annuity plans and senior consideration programs. Individuals depend on these administrations for longer periods as individuals live longer, hence adjustments are expected to ensure they keep on working.

5. Intergenerational Value: The issue of intergenerational value is getting more consideration as it is feasible for more established ages to get more prominent advantages from social and taxpayer driven organizations, possibly to the detriment of more youthful ages who should bear the monetary weight.

6. Wellbeing Disparity: While certain individuals live sound, dynamic lives very much into their senior years, others face serious medical problems. With longer futures comes a significantly more prominent need to address wellbeing aberrations and assurance of impartial admittance to medical services.

7. Moral and Philosophical Issues: The moral ramifications of over the top lifetime expansion, the conveyance of life-augmentation innovation, and the ramifications for individual personality, satisfaction, and design are totally raised by life span.

8. Natural Effect: A populace with a more drawn out life expectancy might overburden the climate and regular assets, in this manner heightening worries about manageability, asset portion, and environmental change.

9. Mechanical Turns of events: New advancements in biotechnology, hereditary qualities, and clinical innovation might assist with people carrying on with longer lives. These progressions hold both expectation and moral problems, for example, how to circulate life-expansion treatments and the implications of overpopulation reasonably.

10. Social and Social Changes: Longer life expectancies can adjust society's standards and convictions, impacting assumptions for retirement ages, family designs, and occupation ways. Foundations inside culture and society should acclimate to these changes.

Numerous states, associations, and researchers are exploring strategies and ways of managing the challenges and potential open doors got on by an ascent life span because of these concerns. To guarantee that more extended lives are quantitatively longer as well as subjectively better and more libertarian, these drives habitually utilize a multidisciplinary approach, consolidating medical care, financial matters, social strategy, and morals. A convoluted and progressing cultural issue that needs cautious thinking and planning on a worldwide level is

adjusting the benefits and hindrances of life
span.

I. What longer futures mean for medical services and society

Future has expanded in numerous locales of the
world because of enhancements in medical care,
sustenance, and day to day environments.
Although longer life expectancies are regularly
viewed as something to be thankful for, they
likewise present open doors and hardships for
medical services frameworks and society at
large. Think about the accompanying significant
variables:

1. Expanded Medical services Expenses:
Ongoing infections and age-related afflictions
like coronary illness, diabetes, and dementia are
regularly more pervasive as life expectancies

increment. In view of the ceaseless clinical consideration and treatment these issues require, medical services costs have developed. Accordingly, medical care frameworks are under strain and may have to go through change to stay reasonable.

2. Senior Consideration: As individuals live longer, there is a rising interest for senior consideration administrations, like nursing homes, assisted residing offices, and home medical services. This presents possibilities for the medical care area yet in addition raises doubt about the availability and cost of such administrations.

3. Rethinking Retirement: Retirement is being rethought because of longer life expectancies. Now that the standard retirement age has been reached, many individuals are contemplating proceeding to work or beginning a subsequent calling. Government backed retirement and annuity projects will be influenced by this.

4. Intergenerational Elements: The elements between ages can be adjusted by longer life expectancies. There might be more interest for more youthful ages to give monetary and providing care backing to their old guardians and grandparents. This might influence relational peculiarities and monetary preparation.

5. Monetary Ramifications: By expanding the quantity of years that a populace is useful, a more extended lived labor force can advance monetary development. In any case, it likewise requires alterations to work markets, including retraining more seasoned specialists, considering adaptable plans for getting work done, and battling age segregation.

Longer life expectancies are a main impetus behind medical services development, remembering headways for medications, innovations, and conveyance frameworks. The improvement of medicines and medications to address the specific wellbeing concerns looked by a maturing populace is a developing area of exploration and medical services supplier consideration.

7. Preventive Medical services: As individuals live longer, preventive medical care turns out to be more significant. It is possible to reduce the weight of ongoing illnesses and save medical care uses by empowering solid ways of life, routine screenings, and early infection conclusion.

8. Social Administrations: Longer life expectancies could require more subsidizing for social administrations including long haul care protection, government managed retirement, and drives to forestall senior depression and segregation.

9. Moral and Legitimate Contemplations: The arrangement of end-of-life care, the dispersion of assets for matured medical services, and advance orders all raise moral issues. To represent the moving demography, lawful designs, and arrangements should change.

10. Personal satisfaction: Eventually, the impacts of longer life expectancies on society ought to be evaluated with regards to both amount and personal satisfaction. It means quite a bit to put forth attempts to ensure that people can live longer, better lives.

For medical services frameworks and society, longer life expectancies are both a test and an open door. It will be important to get ready ahead, put resources into medical care and social administrations, and rethink cultural standards and assumptions encompassing maturing and retirement to adjust to these segment shifts. Longer life expectancies can, in any case, bring about more joyful, better lives for individuals along with further developing society overall with the right arrangements and advances.

B. The Standard Clinical Way to deal with Maturing

The traditional way to deal with medication and maturing involves the utilization of standard operations, drug mediations, and medical care methodologies to fulfill the wellbeing and prosperity prerequisites of maturing individuals. This technique is established on the information that as individuals become more seasoned, they become more inclined to different medical issues and persistent ailments, and that dealing with these hardships requires clinical consideration. Coming up next are a fundamental parts of the conventional way to deal with maturing and medication:

1. Illness The board: In the customary methodology, the fundamental accentuation is much of the time on the determination and therapy of specific ailments and clinical problems every now and again connected to maturing, similar to coronary illness, diabetes, osteoarthritis, and dementia. To treat these illnesses, medical services suppliers utilize different indicative procedures and medicine.

2. Preventive Consideration: Conventional medication additionally underlines playing it safe to bring down the possibility of creating age-related diseases. Normal check-ups, inoculations, tests, and way of life changes remembering guidance for nourishment and exercise are all important for this.

3. Medication: Drugs are a vital part in overseeing age-related medical conditions. Medications might be regulated to patients to oversee torment, decline cholesterol, control pulse, or treat other clinical issues. Due to possible corporations and pessimistic impacts, the utilization of many medications, or polypharmacy, can be tricky in more established people.

4. Surgery: At the point when vital, surgeries are utilized to treat specific ailments. Joint substitutions, waterfall medical procedure, and cardiovascular medical procedure are as often as possible performed on more established patients.

5. Rehabilitation: To help more established people in recuperating from tasks or overseeing constant sicknesses that impede their portability and day to day working, recovery administrations, like non-intrusive treatment and word related treatment, are regularly utilized.

6. Geriatric Consideration: Geriatric medication is a specialty that spotlights on the specific medical care necessities of more seasoned people. Seniors can get exhaustive treatment from geriatricians, who are prepared to address the social, mental, and actual impacts of maturing.

7. Palliative and End-of-Life Care: Conventional medication additionally offers palliative and end-of-life care to the people who are adapting to dangerous sicknesses or are approaching the finish of their lives. These projects work to upgrade living quality, control side effects, and proposition consistent encouragement.

8. Innovative work: Continuous regular clinical exploration looks at novel treatments, meds, and mechanical headways pointed toward improving the wellbeing and prosperity of senior residents. To assess the viability and wellbeing of novel treatments, clinical preliminaries habitually incorporate old people.

9. Medical coverage: Health care coverage frameworks in numerous countries, similar to Federal medical insurance in the US, cover medical services administrations for seniors, making it simpler and more efficient for seniors to get medical care.

It's memorable essential that, despite the fact that the ordinary way to deal with medication and maturing has taken critical steps in expanding and working on the personal satisfaction for more established grown-ups, there is likewise developing acknowledgment of the meaning of reciprocal and elective methodologies, way of life changes, and all encompassing medical services to address the particular requirements of maturing people. A more incorporated technique that blends customary medication with elective wellbeing modalities is being explored by numerous seniors and medical care experts for cultivating general prosperity as individuals age.

I.Healthcare that is illness centered

Sickness focused medical care, some of the time alluded to as the infection focused model or the biomedical model, is a traditional strategy for giving medical services that puts a weighty accentuation on the distinguishing proof and the executives of specific diseases or infirmities. For a significant piece of the twentieth hundred years, this worldview ruled medical care, and it is still vigorously used in contemporary medication. Here are a few fundamental qualities and principles of an illness focused way to deal with medical services:

1. Analysis and Treatment: In this worldview, the fundamental goal is to analyze the specific illness or condition that the patient is experiencing, and afterward to offer particular therapies to diminish or fix the affliction. The underlying driver of a patient's side effects is found out by clinical experts utilizing demonstrative instruments, testing, and clinical information.

2. Specialization: The treatment of infections is regularly joined by the specialization of medical services experts. Zeroing in on specific ailments or organ frameworks are specialists, specialists, radiologists, pathologists, and different subject matter experts. With this specialization, one can treat specific diseases with inside and out information and capability.

3. Drug Intercessions: Medications and drug intercessions are critical to the conveyance of illness centered treatment. Drug remedies from clinical experts are every now and again given to treat diseases, control side effects, or stop the movement of ongoing illnesses.

4. Proof Based Medication: The dynamic cycle in illness focused medical care is exceptionally impacted by logical exploration and proof based medication. To decide the wellbeing and adequacy of drugs, clinical preliminaries, and exploration are utilized.

5. Intense Consideration: Resolving intense clinical issues or crises is ideal for the illness focused model. It represents considerable authority in conveying quick and designated mediations to safeguard life or treat difficult sicknesses or wounds.

6. Momentary Concentration: This model oftentimes gives transient drives the most noteworthy need to address critical wellbeing challenges. It may not necessarily put areas of strength for an on wellbeing advancement or manage the fundamental reasons for clinical issues.

7. Divided Care: Illness focused medical services may periodically bring about divided care, in which a few experts focus on discrete features of a patient's well being without considering the general picture.

Despite the fact that illness focused medical services has demonstrated very powerful in recognizing and treating many clinical issues, it has additionally experienced harsh criticism for certain reasons:

1. Disregarding deterrent Consideration: It probably won't put sufficient accentuation on safeguard endeavors to bring down the event of infections, for example, dietary changes and general wellbeing efforts.

2. Persistent Sickness The board: On account of long haul issues like diabetes and coronary illness, a sickness focused procedure could neglect to address the fundamental way of life factors that cause these issues.

3. High Medical services costs: Treating and practicing generally could bring about high medical services costs, especially while overseeing mind boggling or constant problems.

There has been a change lately toward more understanding focused and all encompassing medical services conveyance models that consider the therapy of diseases as well as the general prosperity of individuals. Preventive consideration, way of life changes, and an emphasis on persistent inclinations and convictions are habitually integrated into these ways to convey more careful and individualized medical services.

Ii. The prerequisite for a change in outlook

As our general public arrangements with the advantages and difficulties welcomed on by a maturing populace, the requirement for a worldview change in life span is turning out to be increasingly self-evident. The expansion of human life span is a convoluted and different point that requires an adjustment of our mentalities, activities, and guidelines. A change in outlook in life expectancy is expected for the accompanying reasons:

1. Segment Shift: A few countries are going through a segment change as the extent of old individuals rises. We should reevaluate how we support and cooperate with more seasoned individuals because of this pattern, which puts tension on medical care frameworks, benefits assets, and social administrations.

2. Healthspan versus Life expectancy: The objective ought to be to live better, more useful lives over a more extended period instead of just to live longer. Expanded wellbeing range, or broadening how much time without persistent sicknesses and handicaps, ought to be the essential objective of a worldview change in life span.

3. Financial Maintainability: As people live longer, the conventional retirement model couldn't be reasonable from a monetary outlook. To protect monetary dependability, we really want to reconsider retirement ages, retirement reserve funds, and more seasoned specialists' commitment to the labor force.

4. Medical care Advancement: A change in outlook animates financing for drives in medical care and exploration about maturing related illnesses. Propels in modified medication, protection measures, and regenerative medication are remembered for this.

5. Social Consideration: Social prohibition and bias against more established individuals are regular events. Advancing intergenerational connections, local area contribution, and social consideration are key parts of moving the worldview in light of the fact that they assist with making people feel associated and deliberate.

6. Strategy and Arranging: States and associations should adjust their arrangements and procedures to represent the moving demography. This involves building age-accommodating metropolitan regions, thinking of long haul care arrangements, and handling issues like senior maltreatment and disregard.

7.Change in Social and Disposition: It's fundamental to adjust how society respects maturing. The colossal commitments more seasoned individuals can provide for society through their experience, information, and gifts ought to be perceived instead of being viewed as a weight.

8. Moral Contemplations: As we increment the typical lifetime of individuals, moral quandaries arise about subjects like asset circulation, end-of-life care, and the chance of overpopulation. These ethical problems request cautious consideration before a change in perspective.

9. Innovative Reconciliation: Embracing innovation can assist more established individuals with carrying on with better lives. This covers drives for computerized consideration as well as the production of savvy home innovation and telemedicine.

10. Lifespan and the Climate: As longer life expectancies can prompt higher asset utilization and ecological pressure, lifespan has natural repercussions. Dependable utilization and manageability ought to be considered in a change in perspective.

The perplexing open doors and challenges presented by a maturing populace are driving the requirement for a change in outlook in life span. It requires a complete technique that considers everything from medical services to financial matters to culture to morals. By reexamining our opinion on maturing, we might make society one in which people live longer, better, and additional delightful lives while resolving the specific issues welcomed on by a maturing populace.

Chapter 2

The Study of Lifespan

The investigation of life span, usually known as gerontology, is a multidisciplinary field devoted to understanding the factors that add to carrying on with a long and solid life. It includes various areas of science, medication, hereditary qualities, way of life, and natural factors that impact the maturing system. The focal objectives of life span science are to expand the human life expectancy and work on personal satisfaction in advanced age. Here are a few huge areas of exploration and variables that add to how we might interpret life span:

1. Genetics: Hereditary factors have an essential part in deciding a singular's life span. Analysts have found specific qualities connected to life expectancy and age-related messes. The hereditary qualities of seemingly perpetual people (centenarians) can uncover bits of knowledge into the hereditary groundwork of life span.

2. Telomeres: Telomeres are the defensive covers at the finishes of chromosomes that abbreviate as cell partition. Telomere shortening has been connected to maturing and age-related messes. Telomere support and expansion is a hotly debated issue in life span science.

3. Cell Senescence: Cell senescence is a condition of irreversible cell cycle capture that is related with maturing and age-related messes. Understanding how to defer or switch cell senescence is a significant subject of study.

4. Caloric Limitation: Lessening calorie consumption without unhealthiness has been found to increase life expectancy in an assortment of taxa, including mice and a few nonhuman primates. Analysts are researching the mechanics of this impact and whether it could be applied to people.

5. Hormonal Elements: Chemicals, for example, development chemical, insulin-like development factor 1 (IGF-1), and sex chemicals impact the maturing system. Chemical substitution treatment and intercessions to advance chemical levels are concentrated on subjects.

6. Diet and Nourishment: An even and nutritious eating routine can significantly affect wellbeing and life span. Diets, for example, the Mediterranean eating routine and discontinuous fasting have been connected to further developed wellbeing results and delayed life expectancy.

7. Exercise: Normal actual work has been related with a lower hazard of constant infections and an improved lifetime. Practice advances strong mass, cardiovascular wellbeing, and generally prosperity.

8. Social and Mental Variables: Life span is connected to social ties, mental prosperity, and a feeling of direction throughout everyday life. Positive social contacts and a solid mental state can assist you with carrying on with a more extended and better life.

9. Against Maturing Treatments: Scientists are exploring a few enemies of maturing mediations, for example, senolytics (drugs that target senescent cells), foundational microorganism treatments, and hereditary designing, to increment life span and further develop wellbeing in advanced age.

Natural components like poisons, contamination, and radiation can all rush the maturing system. It is basic for life expectancy to restrict openness to possibly harming natural impacts.

11. Medical care and Preventive Medication: Approaching quality medical care, normal check-ups, and preventive measures, for example, inoculations can assist you with carrying on with a more extended and better life by overseeing and forestalling illnesses.

12. Customized Medication: Fitting medical care intercessions to a person's hereditary creation, way of life, and wellbeing history can further develop wellbeing and life expectancy results.

While a huge headway has been made in grasping the study of life span, getting critical lifetime expansion in people remains a complicated and changing subject of study. Many elements collaborate to impact a singular's life expectancy, and exploration keeps on uncovering new bits of knowledge and novel intercessions to advance solid maturing and upgrade human life span.

A. Innate Variables and Improvement

Genetic elements assume a significant part in development. While developing is a confounding and complex communication brought about by an assortment of biological, way of life, and innate variables, acquired qualities can essentially impact how individuals age. The following are a couple of basic focuses to consider in regards to hereditary factors and development:

1. Gained Innate Assortments: Our DNA conveys qualities that encode proteins and different substances connected with fundamental normal activities. Genetic varieties, including as single nucleotide polymorphisms (SNPs) and modifications, could impact how these cycles work and, therefore, how an individual develops.

2. Telomeres: Telomere shortening is a sign of development, and when telomeres become basically short, cells might in all likelihood at no point ever segment in the future, bringing about cell development and tissue misfire. Certain individuals have longer or harder telomeres, which can slow the cycle.

3. DNA Fix Frameworks: Our cells have DNA fix parts that assist to keep up with the honesty of our hereditary material. Genetic varieties in DNA fix qualities can impact an individual's repugnance for DNA hurt, which can collect after some time and add to maturing and age-related issues.

4. Mitochondrial DNA: Mitochondria are the forces to be reckoned with of our cells, and they have their own DNA. Changes in mitochondrial DNA can bring about breaking down mitochondria, which can fuel mature-related ailments and lessen generally cell energy yield.

5. hot Responses: Genetic contrasts in disturbance and safe structure highlights can impact an individual's hot response. Steady crabbiness is a side effect of development and has been connected to various age-related illnesses, including cardiovascular infection, diabetes, and neurodegenerative problems.

6. acquired Inclination to Contaminations: A couple of acquired factors increase the gamble of determined age-related messes, like Alzheimer's illness, Parkinson's infection, and a couple of kinds of threatening turn of events. These acquired inclinations can affect an individual's general prosperity and future.

7. Future credits: Specialists have found unequivocal characteristics connected with the future. These qualities might safeguard against age-related issues and add to a more drawn out, better life. FOXO3 quality, for instance, is connected to a higher future in certain populaces.

8. Quality Environment Coordinated efforts: It is basic to stress that hereditary factors don't work alone. They cooperate with normal and way of life components like food, actual work, and noxiousness receptivity to impact the developing framework. This exchange may be complicated and dynamic.

9. Epigenetics: Epigenetic modifications, which can be impacted by both heredity and climate, assume a part in development. changes in DNA methylation, histone adjustments, and non-coding RNA can all influence quality explanation and add to development related modifications.

While innate variables can impact how individuals age and their vulnerability to explicit age-related conditions, it's essential that way of life decisions like a sound eating routine, ordinary activity, and keeping away from hurtful propensities like smoking and inordinate alcohol utilize all fundamentally affect developing. The blend of acquired qualities and way of life conditions is basic in deciding an individual's general prosperity and future. Moreover, stream research in the subject of developing genetic characteristics keeps on uncovering new bits of knowledge into how characteristics impact the developing framework and exceptional medicines to advance strong development.

I. Figuring out the Job of Hereditary qualities in Life span

The impact of hereditary qualities on life expectancy is an intricate and different subject.

Life span, or the possibility to carry on with a more drawn out and better life, is influenced by a blend of hereditary, natural, and social factors. While hereditary qualities really do have an influence, they are just a single component of the jigsaw.

Here are a few urgent focuses to figure out about the impact of hereditary qualities on life span:

1. Hereditary Variety: Qualities are the fundamental units of heredity, and changes in our DNA can influence how long we live. A few hereditary polymorphisms are connected with expanded life span, while others might raise the gamble of specific illnesses that could abbreviate life.

2. Family Ancestry: Family ancestry can give knowledge of the possibility to life span. In the event that you have family members who lived long, sound lives, this might show a hereditary penchant to life span. In any case, it is crucial to understand that hereditary qualities alone don't foresee life expectancy.

3. Life span Qualities: A few individual qualities have been recognized as possibly impacting life span. For instance, the FOXO3 quality has been connected to longer life expectancies in a few populaces. Individual qualities, then again, have a little effect and interface with different variables.

4. Heritability: Heritability alludes to the extent of variety in a variable (for this situation, life expectancy) that is because of hereditary elements. As per studies, hereditary qualities might represent 20-30% of change in human life expectancy, with the equilibrium of variety connected with natural and way of life factors.

5. Quality Climate Connection: Hereditary qualities and climate cooperate to influence life span. People with hereditary inclinations to specific wellbeing problems, for instance, may carry on with longer lives in the event that they embrace a sound way of life and really control their gambling factors.

6. Epigenetics: Epigenetic factors, which involve changes in quality articulation without influencing the basic DNA grouping, can likewise impact life span. Way of life and ecological elements can impact epigenetic changes, affecting quality capability and possibly life expectancy.

7. Normal Life span highlights: A few normal elements associated with life span incorporate keeping a sound body weight, successive actual work, a fair eating regimen, not smoking, moderate liquor admission, and stress the executives. These way of life elements can interface with hereditary qualities to decide life expectancy.

8. Centenarians and Blue Zones: Investigations of centenarians (individuals who live to 100 or past) and "Blue Zones" (locales with high centralizations of enduring people) have featured the significance of way of life, social associations, and diet in life span, even among those with hereditary inclinations.

Hereditary qualities really do play a part in laying out a singular's ability for life span, yet they are just a single part of the situation. Natural and way of life factors, similar to sustenance, exercise, and social ties, significantly affect how long and well we live. Understanding the confounded exchange among hereditary qualities and different variables is basic for empowering great maturing and dragging out life expectancy.

Ii. Hereditary penchant to progress in years related messes

Hereditary inclinations play a critical impact in the improvement of old enough related messes.

These problems are regularly impacted by a blend of hereditary, ecological, and way of life factors. Here are a few instances old enough related messes and the hereditary inclinations to them:

1. Alzheimer's Sickness: Hereditary qualities can affect Alzheimer's sickness. Variations in various qualities, including APOE (Apolipoprotein E), TREM2 (Setting off Receptor Communicated on Myeloid Cells 2), and PSEN1 (Presenilin 1), have been connected with an expanded gamble of Alzheimer's illness. People with specific APOE hereditary varieties, like APOE4, are at an expanded gamble of gaining the condition.

2. Coronary illness: A few genetic factors can expand the gamble of coronary illness, including coronary conduit sickness and hypertension. Varieties in qualities connected with cholesterol digestion, blood coagulating, and vein capability can all add to a singular's powerlessness to coronary illness.

3. Type 2 Diabetes: While way of life factors, for example, food and exercise are significant in the improvement of type 2 diabetes, heredity likewise assumes a part. Variations in qualities like TCF7L2 (Record Element 7-Like 2) have been connected to an expanded gamble of type 2 diabetes.

4. Osteoporosis: Osteoporosis, a problem described by fragile and powerless bones, can have a hereditary part. Variations in qualities related with bone thickness control and collagen development can change a singular's weakness to osteoporosis.

5. Cancer: Many sorts of malignant growth become more normal as people age and genetic variables could build a singular's gamble. Changes in specific qualities, like BRCA1 and BRCA2 for bosom and ovarian malignant growth, or APC for colorectal disease, can decisively expand the gamble of getting these tumors.

6. Parkinson's Infection: Hereditary variables play a part in Parkinson's sickness, with transformations in qualities like LRRK2 (Leucine-Rich Recurrent Kinase 2) and SNCA (Alpha-Synuclein) expanding the gamble. Nonetheless, by far most of Parkinson's cases are irregular and not straightforwardly connected to heredity.

7. Age-Related Macular Degeneration (AMD): Hereditary inclination is a critical part in AMD, a main source of vision misfortune in more seasoned people. Variations in qualities like CFH (Supplement Element H) and ARMS2 (Age-Related Maculopathy Defenselessness 2) have been connected to an expanded gamble of AMD.

It is critical to recollect that having a hereditary weakness to an age-related infection doesn't suggest that a singular will foster the condition. Natural variables, way of life decisions (like nourishment, exercise, and smoking), and general wellbeing all assume significant parts in sickness improvement. Hereditary testing and directing can assist individuals with understanding their hereditary gamble factors and settle on informed conclusions about their wellbeing and preventive measures. Besides, proceeding with research keeps on tracking down more about the mind boggling interaction among hereditary qualities and age-related messes, giving possibilities to early location and custom-made treatment.

B. Epigenetics and Maturing

Epigenetics and maturing are two interconnected fields of study that examine how changes in quality articulation and hereditary control add to the maturing system. Epigenetics alludes to changes in quality movement and articulation that don't involve changes to the fundamental DNA succession. All things considered, epigenetic adjustments involve substance changes to DNA and related proteins, for example, histones, which can impact how qualities are turned on or off.

This is the way epigenetics connects with the maturing system:

1. DNA Methylation: One of the most well-informed epigenetic modifications related to maturing is DNA methylation. Methylation is the expansion of a methyl gathering to specific cytosine bases in DNA. Age-related varieties in DNA methylation designs have been found, for certain qualities turning out to be more methylated (quieted) and others turning out to be less methylated (enacted) as we age. This can influence quality articulation and add to mature-related illnesses.

2. Histone Alterations: Histones are proteins that guide the bundling and consolidating of

DNA into a minimized construction known as chromatin. Different synthetic changes, like acetylation and methylation, can happen on histones, adjusting DNA openness to record factors and other administrative proteins. Changes in histone alterations can impact quality articulation and add to maturing-related side effects.

3. Non-Coding RNAs: Non-coding RNAs, including microRNAs and long non-coding RNAs, have a capability in quality articulation guidelines. These RNA atoms can tie to courier RNAs (mRNAs) and either upgrade or impede their interpretation into proteins. Dysregulation of non-coding RNAs has been connected to maturing and age-related illnesses.

4. Telomere Shortening: Telomeres are rehashed DNA groupings at the finishes of chromosomes that defend them from debasement. Telomeres normally abbreviate with every cell division, and when they develop excessively short, cells could enter senescence or pass on (apoptosis). Epigenetic modifications can impact the speed of telomere shortening and cell maturing.

5. Epigenetic Tickets: Scientists have built epigenetic tickers because of exceptional DNA methylation designs that can decide an individual's natural age. These timekeepers utilize epigenetic changes in an individual's DNA to gauge their age, which can then measure up to their sequential age. Deviations from the projected age might show sped-up or eased-back maturing.

6. Ecological Elements: Epigenetic changes can be impacted by various natural elements, including diet, way of life, harmful openness, and stress. These elements can either speed up or slow the maturing system by affecting epigenetic changes.

Understanding the connection between epigenetics and maturing is basic for uncovering the sub-atomic components behind maturing and age-related illnesses. It additionally gives potential ways for treatments to advance solid maturing and increment life span by focusing on epigenetic changes. Notwithstanding, a huge examination is as yet being directed regarding this matter, and many worries about the exact systems engaged with the epigenetic guideline of maturing stay inexplicable.

I..How way of life and natural variables influence the nature of enunciation

A trademark known as epigenetics permits way of life and ecological elements to extensively affect the nature of verbalization. Rather than changes in the DNA arrangement itself, epigenetics alludes to changes in quality verbalization that are welcomed by changes to the DNA molecule or the proteins related with it. Here are a few instances of how changes in the way of life and natural impacts could influence the nature of verbalization:

1. DNA Methylation: Methylation is the most common way of changing a substance and includes pressing a methyl bunch inside a DNA molecule. Methylation commonly brings about quiet quality, which proposes that the quality is more averse to be created. Diet, smoking, and weakness to normal poisons are a couple of the elements that could influence DNA methylation designs. For instance, a high-fat eating regimen has been connected to expanded DNA methylation in obvious ways, which might add to the movement of illnesses like stoutness and diabetes.

2. Histone Alterations: Proteins called histones are liable for sorting out and packaging DNA inside cells. Histones can go through fake adjustments like acetylation and methylation, which can influence how firmly the DNA is folded over the histones and thus influence the nature of explanation. Histone alterations and, thus, the nature of explanation can be impacted by pressure, diet, and receptiveness to regular pollutants.

3. Non-Coding RNAs: By restricting themselves to courier RNA (mRNA) particles and either helping or hindering these atoms' interpretation into proteins, non-coding RNAs, as microRNAs and long non-coding RNAs, can affect the nature of protein explanation. These non-coding RNAs are helpless to a scope of ecological and way of life factors, including dietary admission and defenselessness to disease.

4. Sustenance and Diet: An individual's eating routine hugely affects how well they can explain. The capacity to record factors, histone alterations, and DNA methylation can be in every way affected by enhancements and dietary fixings. For example, a B nutrient called folate is fundamental for ordinary DNA methylation and its need might bring about change in quality explanation plans.

5. Exercise: By changing the development of different record parts and hailing channels, standard genuine work can influence the nature of explanation. The training has been displayed to influence qualities connected areas of strength for to, irritation, and absorption.

6. Stress: By delivering pressure particles like cortisol, relentless strain can change the nature of enunciation. These hormonal modifications might influence the qualities associated with pressure responses, invulnerability, and other physiological cycles.

7. Environmental Toxins: Openness to natural poisons like contamination, weighty metals, and engineered mixtures might result in epigenetic changes that influence the lucidity of discourse. For example, tobacco use can adjust the examples of DNA methylation in lung cells, expanding the gamble of cell breakdown in the lungs.

8. Aging: Quality enunciation plans change as we age. Over the long haul, epigenetic changes compound, bringing about changes in the manner in which the body puts itself out there as it ages.

It is basic to underline that these epigenetic changes can some of the time be switched. A smart dieting routine, predictable activity, and stretching the boundaries can assist with reducing a portion of the impeding effects of natural impacts on the nature of discourse. Figuring out the perplexing communication between acquired qualities, epigenetics, and natural/way of life factors is a consistent subject of examination with proposals for wellbeing and infection counteraction.

II. The Chance of Epigenetic Treatments

Epigenetic treatments are effectively being explored for various afflictions and sicknesses and propositions significantly expected in the space of prosperity. The expression "epigenetics" alludes to changes in quality verbalization or cell total that do exclude adjustments to the basic DNA structure however are rather interceded by changes to DNA and histone proteins. These movements can be turned around, which makes them convincing contenders for successful intervention. The following are a couple of unmistakable regions where epigenetic drugs have shown viability:

1. Treatment for dangerous development: The beginning and movement of dangerous development are generally affected by epigenetic changes. Certain malignancies, for example, myelodysplastic conditions and cutaneous lymphocyte lymphoma, have been endorsed for treatment with epigenetic drugs, for example, DNA methyltransferase inhibitors, (for example, 5-azacytidine) and histone deacetylase inhibitors, (for example, vorinostat). These drugs have the ability to reestablish atypical DNA methylation and histone adjustments, reactivate development silencer properties, and defer the beginning of sickness.

2. Neurological Issues: Epigenetic modifications have been connected to neurodegenerative illnesses like Alzheimer's and Parkinson's as well as neurodevelopmental issues like Rett's disorder. By zeroing in on clear epigenetic markings related with different illnesses, experts are examining epigenetic treatments to reduce or fix contamination development possibly.

3. Phenomenal Inherited Infections: A few interesting innate illnesses, for example, Prader-

Willi condition and Angelman problem, are brought about by various quality etching welcomed on by epigenetic changes. Potential medicines incorporate epigenetic drugs that focus on the unmistakable attributes related with specific illnesses.

4. Cardiovascular Illness: Hypertension and atherosclerosis are two cardiovascular infections that are connected with epigenetic changes. Scientists are investigating epigenetic treatments to further develop discourse quality and lessen the gamble factors related with specific illnesses.

5. Red hot and Resistant Framework Contaminations: By zeroing in on attributes related with irritation and the safe framework, epigenetic medicines might assist with changing how the body answers illnesses like lupus and rheumatoid joint torment.

6. Life length and development: Epigenetic adjustments are related to maturational cycles. To revamp cells and perhaps protract sound life, a few scientists are investigating epigenetic treatments like senolytic drugs.

7. Regenerative Medication: Epigenetic adjustments are significant for the recuperation of tissue and the division of undifferentiated cells. The advancement of regenerative meds can profit from a comprehension of and the board of these epigenetic marks.

8. Redone Medicine: By recognizing explicit epigenetic alterations connected to illness chance or movement, epigenetic profiling of individual patients might support modifying treatment regimens. This might bring about additional exact and strong prescriptions.

Regardless of its enormous responsibility, epigenetic treatments are not without hindrances and possible downsides. Off-target impacts, long stretch security, and the requirement for individualized drugs are a couple of the difficulties that should be tended to in the course and arranging of epigenetic medicines.

Furthermore, more exploration is expected to all the more likely comprehend the complex epigenetic components of numerous illnesses and to further develop treatment choices. By and by, the potential for epigenetic therapies to change clinical consideration and give new supportive answers for a large number of issues is a captivating and extending subject of study.

C, The Capability of Telomeres

Telomeres are fundamental in cell science, especially in the support of genomic steadiness and the guideline of cell lifetime. These particular DNA successions are situated at the finishes of direct chromosomes in eukaryotic cells, including human cells. Telomeres assume the accompanying basic parts:

1. Chromosome Insurance: Telomeres work as defensive covers at the closures of chromosomes. Their rehashed groupings and related proteins keep the typical closures of chromosomes from being recognized as DNA harm. This protection keeps chromosomes fundamentally in one piece and keeps them from combining or debasing.

2. DNA Replication: During cell division, DNA is replicated so every little girl cell gets a total supplement of hereditary data. Notwithstanding, because of its limitations, the DNA replication hardware can't completely duplicate the actual closures of direct chromosomes. Telomeres go about as a cushion zone, permitting rehashed rounds of cell division without impressive loss of basic hereditary material.

3. Cell Life Expectancy Guideline: Telomeres are habitually contrasted with cell clocks. Telomeres are abbreviated as cell isolates because of insufficient DNA replication at the closures of chromosomes. At the point when telomeres get perilously short, cells enter a state known as senescence, which is a sort of irreversible cell cycle stop. This technique means to forestall the uncontrolled division of harmed or possibly dangerous cells.

4. Maturing and Illness: Telomere length is connected to the maturing system. Telomeres are persistently abbreviated as cells in our bodies partition all through our lives. At the point when telomeres become excessively short, cells become less useful, bringing about the physical and practical crumbling related to maturing.

Telomere shortening has likewise been related to various age-related illnesses, including malignant growth, cardiovascular illness, and neurological issues.

5. Cell Interminability: In contrast to substantial cells, certain cells, like foundational microorganisms and microbe cells, have systems that permit them to keep up with or even extend their telomeres. This allows these cells to gap and make new cells continually, helping with tissue fix and generation. Telomerase, a protein that can stretch telomeres, is dynamic in these cells however is regularly curbed in most substantial cells.

Understanding the meaning of telomeres has significant ramifications for maturing research, disease science, and regenerative medication. Specialists are investigating ways of adjusting telomeres and telomerase to possibly stretch cell life span, defer the maturing system, and track down new therapies for age-related problems and malignant growth. Be that as it may, these drives are still in their beginning stages and require extra examination and moral contemplation.

I., Telomere shortening and cell maturing

Telomere shortening is a characteristic organic cycle that is firmly connected to cell maturing. How about we separate the idea to all the more likely understand this association:

1. Telomeres: Telomeres are defensive covers situated at the closures of straight chromosomes in the core of eukaryotic cells (cells with a real core, like human cells). They are composed of rehashed DNA arrangements and related proteins. Their key job is to safeguard the chromosome's honesty by keeping the closures from corrupting or converging with adjoining chromosomes.

2. Cell Division: In generally substantial (body) cells, cell division (mitosis) is fundamental for tissue development, recuperation, and upkeep. At the point when a cell partitions, the DNA is copied, yet because of how DNA replication happens, a little piece of the telomere is lost. This is because the replication apparatus failed to copy the outrageous finishes of the chromosomes completely.

3. Telomere Shortening: Telomeres abbreviate with each round of cell division. This shortening becomes recognizable over the long run. At the point when telomeres get seriously short, they can never again safeguard the chromosome and the cell enters a state known as **senescence**.

4. Cell Maturing: Cell senescence is an irreversible cell cycle stop. Cells in this state can never again separate and add to tissue fix and support. This is an indication of maturing in tissues and organs, and it has been associated with a few age-related messes.

5. Telomerase: In certain phones, like microorganism cells (sperm and egg cells) and undifferentiated organisms, a protein called telomerase might broaden telomeres, permitting these phones to isolate a few times without telomere shortening. For this reason, microbe cells might give hereditary material from one age to another without causing significant telomere harm. Be that as it may, most physical cells have somewhat low amounts of telomerase, which adds to telomere shortening and cell maturing.

6. Illness and Maturing: Telomere shortening is connected to an expanded gamble of old enough related illnesses like cardiovascular infection, diabetes, and certain types of disease. While telomere shortening adds to maturing, it isn't the essential indicator of a singular's life span. Hereditary qualities, way of life factors, and other natural cycles all assume significant parts.

Telomeres and telomerase are being read up as imminent focuses for treatments that could dial back cell maturing or treat age-related diseases. Be that as it may, it is a convoluted area of exploration, and substantially more should be advanced before such arrangements become comprehensively accessible. In the meantime, keeping a solid way of life through food, exercise, and stress the board can assist with easing back the maturing system and improving cell well-being.

II., Telomere length safeguarding techniques

Supporting telomere length is basic for supporting cell well-being and possibly diminishing the maturing system. Telomeres are defensive covers at the closures of chromosomes that are normally abbreviated as cell partition. At the point when telomeres become excessively short, cells can become senescent or bite the dust, which can prompt maturing and age-related messes. While you can't stay away from telomere shortening, you can utilize way of life ways of behaving to assist with protecting telomere length and backing general well-being:

1. Eat an even eating regimen high in cell reinforcements, nutrients, and minerals. Cell reinforcements assist with safeguarding cells from oxidative pressure, which can hurry telomere shortening. Lean proteins, entire grains, organic products, and veggies are incredible choices.

2. Getting Sufficient Rest: Hold back nothing long periods of good rest every evening. Rest is fundamental for cell fix and recovery, which can help with saving telomere length.

3. Normal Activity: - Participate in ordinary actual work, including both vigorous and strength preparation. The practice has been demonstrated to increment telomerase movement, a protein that can protract telomeres.

4. Stress The board: Ongoing pressure could hurry telomere shortening. Use pressure-decrease systems like care contemplation, yoga, profound breathing activities, or loosening up side interests.

5. Keep a Solid Weight: Weight and additional fat can add to aggravation and oxidative pressure, the two of which can disable telomeres. Keeping a sound load with diet and exercise may be worthwhile.

6. Omega-3 Unsaturated fats: Omega-3 unsaturated fats, tracked down in greasy fish, flaxseeds, and pecans, have calming characteristics and may assist with safeguarding telomeres.

7. Limit Sugar and Handled Food varieties: High-sugar and handled food diets could add to aggravation and oxidative pressure. Lessen your utilization of sweet drinks and handled food varieties.

8. Limit Liquor and Smoking: Over-the-top liquor use and smoking could rush telomere shortening. Assuming that you smoke, find support to stop, and restrict or avoid drinking.

9. Remain Hydrated: Drinking sufficient water upholds general cell well-being, which can in a roundabout way help with safeguarding telomere length.

10. Supplements: A few enhancements, like vitamin D, may assist with telomere upkeep.

Before integrating any enhancements into your routine, talk with a medical care master.

11. Keeping up major areas of strength with associations and a supporting organization of loved ones lightens pressure and increments general prosperity.

12. Long-lasting Learning: - Participating in mental exercises and constant learning can help psychological well-being by possibly lessening pressure and supporting telomere conservation.

Recall that hereditary qualities assume a part in telomere length and that not all parts of telomere shortening can be made due. A sound way of life, then again, can assist with decreasing the speed of telomere shortening and add to general well-being and life span. Counsel a medical services expert for customized direction on telomere well-being and maturing issues.

D. New Age-Switching Advances

The field hostile to maturing innovation is expanding rapidly, and innovative work is continuous. As we assess probably the latest enemy of maturing innovations and ideas that are standing out, remember that huge headways might have occurred from that point forward. The following are a couple of prominent areas of hostility to maturing study and development:

1. Senolytics: Senescent cells, which collect with maturing and play a part in a few age-related illnesses, are cells that are quite isolating. Medicine or different medications known as senolytics target and kill these cells. Research in this space is as yet being finished, and it might assist with forestalling age-related diseases.

2. Telomere extending: Telomeres, which act as chromosome closures' defensive covers, become more limited with maturing. A few examinations searched for ways of keeping up with or extending telomeres to maybe sluggish or quit maturing. In any case, there is still discussion encompassing this issue, hence more exploration is essential.

3. **Nicotinamide adenine dinucleotide (NAD+) supplementation:** As individuals age, their bodies produce less of this atom, which is engaged with a few cell processes. Utilizing forerunners like nicotinamide riboside (NR) or nicotinamide mononucleotide (NMN), a few scientists were exploring NAD+ supplementation as an expected enemy of maturing treatment.

4. **Quality treatment**: New quality-altering procedures like CRISPR-Cas9 have raised the chance of modifying maturing-related qualities to broaden life or defer age-related illnesses. Research was being finished around here.

5. **Undifferentiated cell treatment**: Regenerative medication and hostile to maturing

undifferentiated organism-based treatments have shown guarantee. Undeveloped cells might be utilized to fix harmed tissues and recover organs impacted by maturing, as indicated by research.

6. Caloric limitation and irregular fasting: These dietary practices have shown guarantee in broadening life expectancy and further developing well-being in various model species, and concentrates on caloric limitation and discontinuous fasting were in progress. Scientists were investigating the cycles that underlie these impacts.

Inhibitors of the Senescence-Related Secretory Aggregate (SASP): Senescent cells show the SASP, in which they discharge poisonous mixtures into the tissue around them. A piece of hostility to maturing research has been committed to making drugs that will diminish SASP.

8. The epigenetic clock and epigenetic restoration: Researchers are attempting to comprehend how the epigenome changes as we age and how to switch or return these progressions to a more energetic state.

9. Customized medication: Hostile to maturing treatments that are customized to an individual's hereditary make-up, way of life, and specific maturing-related medical problems are turning out to be more famous. Strategies that are custom-fitted to the individual can yield improved results.

10. Man-made reasoning and AI: Calculations in light of computerized reasoning and AI were utilized to dissect tremendous datasets about maturing and offer novel experiences, possibly prompting the improvement of new enemies of maturing mediations.

Despite the capability of these innovations, hostile to maturing research is a muddled field, and numerous medicines might in any case be in their outset or beginning stages. It is fundamental to counsel medical care experts and uses proof-based rehearses before utilizing any enemy of maturing strategy. The turn of events and utilization of against-maturing advances additionally intensely rely upon moral and administrative issues.

D. New Age-Switching Advances

The field hostile to maturing innovation is expanding rapidly, and innovative work is continuous. As we assess probably the latest enemy of maturing innovations and ideas that are standing out, remember that huge headways might have occurred from that point forward. The following are a couple of prominent areas of hostility to maturing study and development:

1. Senolytics: Senescent cells, which collect with maturing and play a part in a few age-related illnesses, are cells that are quite isolating. Medicine or different medications known as senolytics target and kill these cells. Research in this space is as yet being finished, and it might assist with forestalling age-related diseases.

2. Telomere extending: Telomeres, which act as chromosome closures' defensive covers, become more limited with maturing. A few examinations searched for ways of keeping up with or extending telomeres to maybe sluggish or quit maturing. In any case, there is still discussion encompassing this issue, hence more exploration is essential.

3. Nicotinamide adenine dinucleotide (NAD+) supplementation: As individuals age, their bodies produce less of this atom, which is engaged with a few cell processes. Utilizing forerunners like nicotinamide riboside (NR) or nicotinamide mononucleotide (NMN), a few scientists were exploring NAD+ supplementation as an expected enemy of maturing treatment.

4. Quality treatment: New quality-altering procedures like CRISPR-Cas9 have raised the chance of modifying maturing-related qualities to broaden life or defer age-related illnesses. Research was being finished around here.

5. Undifferentiated cell treatment: Regenerative medication and hostile to maturing undifferentiated organism-based treatments have shown guarantee. Undeveloped cells might be utilized to fix harmed tissues and recover organs impacted by maturing, as indicated by research.

6. Caloric limitation and irregular fasting: These dietary practices have shown guarantee in broadening life expectancy and further developing well-being in various model species, and concentrates on caloric limitation and discontinuous fasting were in progress. Scientists were investigating the cycles that underlie these impacts.

7.Inhibitors of the Senescence-Related Secretory Aggregate (SASP): Senescent cells show the SASP, in which they discharge poisonous mixtures into the tissue around them. A piece of hostility to maturing research has been committed to making drugs that will diminish SASP.

8. The epigenetic clock and epigenetic restoration: Researchers are attempting to comprehend how the epigenome changes as we age and how to switch or return these progressions to a more energetic state.

9. Customized medication: Hostile to maturing treatments that are customized to an individual's hereditary make-up, way of life, and specific maturing-related medical problems are turning out to be more famous. Strategies that are custom-fitted to the individual can yield improved results.

10. Man-made reasoning and AI: Calculations in light of computerized reasoning and AI were utilized to dissect tremendous datasets about maturing and offer novel experiences, possibly prompting the improvement of new enemies of maturing mediations.

Despite the capability of these innovations, hostile to maturing research is a muddled field, and numerous medicines might in any case be in their outset or beginning stages. It is fundamental to counsel medical care experts and uses proof-based rehearses before utilizing any enemy of maturing strategy. The turn of events and utilization of against-maturing advances additionally intensely rely upon moral and administrative issues.

I..Senescence and cell restoration

Senescence and cell restoration are two restricting cycles that assume significant parts in the science of cells and life forms, quite with regards to maturing and tissue recovery. How about we dig further into these thoughts:

1. Senescence: Cell senescence is a condition where a cell loses its capacity to separation and capability regularly. It is regularly connected with maturing and is an ordinary component of the phone cycle.

- DNA harm, telomere shortening, oxidative pressure, and various cell stressors can all add to senescence. Telomeres are the defensive covers on the finishes of chromosomes that abbreviate with every cell division and are much of the time related with cell maturing.

- Senescent cells display specific modifications, like an extended and leveled appearance, expanded discharge of provocative

synthetic compounds (senescence-related secretory aggregate or SASP), and changed quality articulation designs.
- Senescence can be valuable in certain circumstances since it forestalls the improvement of harmed or possibly dangerous cells.
It fills in as a technique to diminish cancer development.
- In any case, an amassing of senescent cells in tissues after some time could prompt age-related illnesses and tissue breakdown, depicted as "senescence-related illnesses."

2. Cell Revival: Cell restoration is the most common way of reestablishing or working on the usefulness and wellbeing of matured or senescent cells. This technique attempts to switch or delay the impacts of senescence and further develop cell practicality.
- Among the methodologies for cell revival are:
a. Telomere expansion: Some exploration attempts to extend telomeres, maybe permitting

cells to keep separating and deferring the beginning of senescence.

b. Senolytics: Senolytic drugs are being created to explicitly target and annihilate senescent cells from tissues, thus bringing down the adverse consequences of senescence-related aggravation.

c. Immature microorganism treatments: Foundational microorganisms can supplant harmed or senescent cells and remake tissues.

d. Hostile to maturing intercessions: Way of life factors like a decent eating regimen, exercise, and stress the board can assist with deferring the maturing system and backing cell wellbeing.

a. Hereditary and epigenetic intercessions: Propels in hereditary designing and epigenetic alteration might give ways of reviving cells at the sub-atomic level.

Endeavors to comprehend and control senescence and cell revival are dynamic review regions in science, regenerative medication, and maturing. A definitive objective is to recognize procedures to expand solid life expectancy, defer age-related messes, and work on the overall personal satisfaction in the old. Be that as it may, while progress has been accomplished, huge obstacles stay in changing these discoveries into feasible clinical medicines for maturing related diseases.

Ii. The Obligation to Regenerative Medication

The commitment to regenerative medication is a spearheading area of exploration and clinical consideration that holds an extraordinary commitment to changing how we approach and treat a large number of diseases, wounds, and clinical issues. Using the body's intrinsic capacity to fix and recover tissues and organs is at the center of regenerative medication. The following are a couple of huge parts of the commitment to regenerative medication:

1. Recuperation of Harmed or Sick Tissues and Organs: Regenerative medication attempts to reestablish or supplant ailing or harmed tissues and organs by helping the body's self-upkeep systems. Various strategies, for example, principal microorganism treatment, tissue planning, and quality treatment, can be utilized to achieve this.

2. Treatment for undifferentiated organic entities: In the human body, undifferentiated cells can form into numerous cell types. They can be applied to reestablish or supplant harmed organs and tissues. Undifferentiated cell treatments can fix illnesses like Parkinson's and Alzheimer's contamination, coronary infection, diabetes, and spinal line wounds.

3. Tissue Planning: In the exploration office, using a mix of cells, biomaterials, and improvement factors, tissue planning is the most well-known strategy for creating fake tissues and organs. Then, patients can get these adjusted tissues to supplant harmed or missing organs. This technique has shown dependability in fields like skin units, tendon fixes, and, amazingly, the creation of phony organs.

4. Quality Treatment: Quality treatment looks to address or supplant defects that outcome in obtained wrecks. Experts might have the option to change or add express credits to a patient's telephone to fix hereditary issues.

5. Custom-fitted Medicine: The idea of a uniquely designed drug is firmly connected with the idea of regenerative medication. Clinical experts can work on the viability of regenerative medicines while decreasing accidental secondary effects and dangers by fitting treatment to an individual's specially acquired beauty care products and clinical history.

6. Less reliance on Organ Moves: Regenerative medication's capacity to decrease dependence on organ transplantation is perhaps its most charming component. Patients could get lab-created organs or tissues matched to their science as opposed to hanging tight for benefactor organs, diminishing the dangers of relocation dismissal and the hardships related to organ deficiency.

7. Treatment for Constant Sickness: Regenerative medication can offer long-haul treatments and even remedies for determined and degenerative ailments for which there is currently no fix, like diabetes, Parkinson's illness, and a few different sorts of problems.

8. Zeroed in on Fix and Recovery:
Regenerative treatments can rush the recuperating system in instances of serious wounds, sports wounds, and business-related wounds. They could bring about speedier recuperation times and improved results for the patients.

9. Moral and managerial issues:
Notwithstanding its colossal potential, regenerative medication faces moral and authoritative issues, for example, guaranteeing the security of preliminary meds, settling worries about genetic adjustment, and laying out rules for the investigation and treatment of youthful microorganisms.

10. Continuous Innovative Work: The field of regenerative medication is continually

expanding because of progressing innovative work. We will no doubt see undifferentiated living beings, hereditary qualities, and tissue plans diversely because of new meds and utilizations.

Regenerative medication can upset the clinical business by giving proficient medicines to a large number of clinical diseases and upgrading the prosperity of incalculable individuals. While impediments to endurance exist, the potential advantages make it a fascinating and alluring region for sensible and clinical examination.

Chapter 3

The Specialty of Lifespan

The methods, customs, and lifestyle that can prompt a more drawn-out and better life are alluded to as the "specialty of life span." The capacity to get medical care, climate, and hereditary qualities are only a couple of the numerous factors that influence life expectancy. To work on their possibilities of carrying on with a more drawn-out and seriously fulfilling existence, individuals can keep a few rules and strategies, including:

Quite possibly the main consideration advancing life span is eating a fair, nutritious eating regimen. Make certain to underline ingesting various natural products, vegetables, entire grains, lean meats, and solid fats. Handled food varieties, improved refreshments, and unnecessary liquor utilization ought to be stayed away from or restricted.

2. Ordinary Activity: Actual work is urgent for saving well-being and expanding life. To keep up with your body vigorous and your cardiovascular framework solid, practice often by strolling, swimming, cycling, or strength preparing.

3. Stress the board: Long-haul pressure can be awful for your well-being. To oversee pressure, attempt pressure-decrease practices like care, yoga, profound breathing, or contemplation.

4. Satisfactory Rest: Life span and general prosperity rely upon getting sufficient rest. To give your body time to retouch and recover, attempt to get somewhere in the range of 7 and 9 hours of sound rest consistently.

5. Social Associations: Having major areas of strength for an organization and a feeling of having a place can increment life span. Invest energy with friends, family and companions in satisfying connections, and partake in pleasant social exercises.

6. Emotional well-being: Put your emotional wellness first by getting the help you want, dealing with yourself, and doing mental-testing leisure activities like perusing, riddles, or learning new things.

7. Stop Smoking: Smoking has been connected to numerous afflictions and can decrease lifetime. There are both present-moment and long-term well-being benefits to stopping smoking.

8. Drink Respectably: An excess of liquor drinking may be unsafe for your well-being. Assuming that you do, use balance while drinking.

9. Plan Ordinary Exams: To recognize and address potential medical problems early, plan routine clinical tests and screenings.

10. Keep Your Psyche occupied: All through your life, keep your brain occupied and intrigued. To do this, you could take part in leisure activities, get new abilities, and keep an interest in the planet.

11. Moderate Caloric Admission: Some exploration shows that calorie limitation without ailing health might protract life expectancy in certain species. The information for individuals, notwithstanding, is less indisputable. Even though it is ordinarily exhorted against gorging for wellbeing, it means a lot to keep a solid weight.

12. Hereditary advising: You might need to seek after hereditary guidance assuming the family has a past filled with specific hereditary illnesses or issues that might abbreviate life ranges. This can assist you with better comprehension of your dangers and empower you to use sound judgment.

13. Ecological Mindfulness: Know about your environmental factors, particularly your openness to poisons and contamination. Stay away from perilous substance openness however much you can.

14. Positivity: Keep an uplifting perspective on life and a bright disposition. A more extended, more joyful life might result from hopefulness and a feeling of direction.

15. Local area Commitment: Partake in your area through charitable efforts or other community exercises. Life span can profit from a feeling of having a place for a more noteworthy reason.

Recall that individual variables and conditions could change, so adjusting these rules to your specific circumstance and looking for the help of medical care experts for custom-fitted direction on further developing longevity is essential. To carry on with a long and solid life as you become more established, you should use sound judgment and go to proactive lengths.

A...Lifestyle factors that influence life span

Your overall well-being and life expectancy are enormously affected by way of life decisions. Regardless of whether hereditary qualities likewise have an effect, driving a solid way of life can significantly work on your possibilities of living a more drawn-out, better life. The following are a couple of fundamental way of life components for life span:

1. Nutrition: Life span relies upon a sound, supplement-rich eating routine. Make certain to underline the consumption of various organic products, vegetables, entire grains, lean meats, and solid fats. Lessen how much handled food varieties, sweet beverages, and inordinate salt you eat.

2. Actual work: Customary actual work gives a few well-being benefits, like bringing down the gamble of constant illnesses, keeping a sound weight, and upgrading cardiovascular well-being. Hold back nothing 75 minutes of demanding movement or 150 minutes of moderate vigorous action each week, alongside strength preparation.

3. Stress the executives: Long-haul pressure can be terrible for your well-being. To oversee pressure, practice pressure-decrease practices like care, yoga, profound breathing, or contemplation.

4. Quality Rest: For a life span, having customary, great quality sleep is fundamental. To give your body time to fix and recuperate, attempt to get somewhere in the range of 7 and 9 hours of solid rest each evening.

5. Social Associations: Having areas of strength for a local area and keeping up major areas of strength with ties can be valuable for your psychological and close-to-home well-being.

The gamble of misery and mental crumbling can be diminished through friendly contribution.

6. Keep away from unsafe propensities: Limit liquor admission and quit smoking. While extreme liquor use can bring about some medical problems, smoking is one of the significant reasons for superfluous passes.

7. Routine Clinical Check-Ups: Routine clinical assessments and screenings can help recognize and oversee medical problems early, improving the probability of fruitful recuperation and long life.

8. Mental Excitement: Keep your psyche dynamic by perusing, addressing puzzles, getting new abilities, or seeking after your innovativeness. As you age, mental excitement can help with keeping up with mental capability.

9. Keep a Sound Weight: Being overweight or stout has been related to an expanded gamble of persistent illnesses like diabetes, coronary illness, and a few kinds of diseases. Through sustenance and exercise, it's vital to reach and keep a sound weight.

10. Appropriate hydration: It is significant for general well-being yet is here and there dismissed. To help various actual frameworks, hydrate every day.

11. Sun Insurance: To bring down your possibilities of skin malignant growth and early maturing, shield your skin from over-the-top sun openness. When required, look for concealment, use sunscreen, and put on defensive stuff.

12. An Uplifting perspective: Keeping an uplifting perspective and a feeling of direction in daily routine will help one experience longer. Invest energy in doing things that make you blissful and fulfilled.

Lessen openness to natural toxic substances and poisons however much as could be expected.

Ensure the spots you live and work energize well-being and security.

Remember that over the long haul, little, reasonable changes to your way of life can hugely affect your overall well-being and life expectancy. A vital part of expanding life span is looking for custom-made counsel from medical care experts.

I..Diet and nourishment are significant primary components.

Without a doubt, significant variables in day-to-day thriving and prosperity are diet and sustenance. For keeping a solid way of life and staying away from various clinical issues, they are fundamental. The following are a couple of vital variables to consider while picking an eating plan and a sustenance plan:

1. Adjusted Diet: A sound eating regimen ought to incorporate different food sources from each dietary class, like natural food varieties, vegetables, entire grains, lean proteins, and dairy items or dairy choices. This gives supplements, minerals, protein, starches, and fats, which are vital parts.

2. Macronutrients: Starches, proteins, and lipids are the three fundamental nourishment classifications in your eating routine.

Each has a particular task to take care of in the body:

- To take care of the body, utilize complex wellsprings of sugars like entire grains, natural food sources, and veggies.

- Proteins are important for the body's safe framework, tissue fix, and a few activities. Lean protein sources incorporate things like tofu, beans, fish, and poultry.

- Even though fats are significant for cell well-being, they ought to come from healthy sources like avocados, almonds, and olive oil.

3. Micronutrients: Even though your body requires a limited quantity of specific supplements and minerals, they are fundamental for ideal well-being. A few models are vitamin D, calcium, iron, and zinc. L-ascorbic corrosive is another. For a fair dietary arrangement, remember these enhancements.

4. Remaining hydrated is fundamental for keeping up with body capabilities. Water is essential for a few cycles, like processing,

course, and managing interior intensity levels
Attempt to hydrate over the day.

5. Portion Control: Watch your segments to
abstain from indulging, which can prompt
weight gain and related dangers to your well-
being.

6. Supplement Timing: Both what and when
you eat may be vital. Attempt to eat continuous
dinners and snacks to keep up with consistent
glucose levels and forestall outrageous appetite.

7. Unmistakable eating designs: Certain
individuals might require exceptional weight-
control systems because of dietary limitations or
one-of-a-kind diseases. A veggie lover or
vegetarian who devours less sugar and dodges
gluten, again and again, gets fitter by eating
fewer calories, which is a model for individuals
with food-responsive qualities, diabetes, and
hypertension.

8. Center around entire, normal eats in any place conceivable to work on dietary quality. Food sources with a great deal of handling and refinement can contain additional sugar, unfortunate fats, and synthetics.

9. Moderation: Appreciate sweets and greasy feast choices with some restraint. While periodically ingesting less animating food sources is satisfactory, you shouldn't base most of your eating routine on them.

10. Counsel a Clinical Consideration Proficient: On the off chance that you have particular ailments or dietary limitations, it is prompted that you counsel an ensured dietitian or a clinical consideration master. They can give suggestions and guidance that explicitly consider your necessities.

It's essential to remember that there is no one size-fits-all way to deal with nourishment. It's conceivable that what turns out splendidly for one individual will not for another. It's urgent to find an eating routine model that upholds your novel well-being goals, eating inclinations and any dynamic clinical worries. Eating a predictable, supplement-rich eating routine and taking part in customary actual work are the most effective ways to improve and keep up with superb well-being all through your life.

Ii. Real action and activities for strong developing

The progression of good development depends energetically upon genuine work and exercise. Supporting a working lifestyle is dire for supporting both physical and mental wellbeing as people age. Contemplate the going with huge nuances:

1.Chipped away at Cardiovascular Prosperity: Typical movement diminishes the risk of cardiovascular disorders and keeps a sound heart. Rehearses that increase cardiovascular health integrate enthusiastic walking, swimming, and cycling.

2. Strength and Balance: Seniors who partake in strength planning rehearsals like weightlifting and obstacle getting ready can stay aware of their bone thickness and solid mass. Besides, offset rehearses help with cutting down the chance of falls, which is a gigantic worry for senior occupants.

3. Joint Prosperity: Exercise can keep joints versatile and cut down the likelihood of encountering joint agony. Joint prosperity is especially redesigned by low-impact practices like yoga .

4. Profound prosperity: Practice deals with mental health by cutting down strain, pressure, and troublesome secondary effects. It can in like manner work on mental capacity and lessen the chance of dementia and age-related mental disintegration.

5. Weight the chiefs: Keeping a strong body weight is critical for thwarting heftiness and its connected ailments, similar to diabetes and hypertension. Weight the chiefs can benefit from standard movement.

6. Social Responsibility: Joining a get-together development or an action class can uphold social affiliation and lessen impressions of melancholy, which are ceaseless in additional laid out individuals.

7. Individual fulfillment: By keeping up a working lifestyle, one can have better real prosperity, compactness, and general success.

The following are a couple of ideas and pointers for incorporating exercise into a sound developing timetable:

- **Chat with a Clinical benefit Capable:** Assuming you have any fundamental prosperity ailments or concerns, it's vital to talk with your clinical benefits expert prior to beginning any exercise plan.

- **Select Tomfoolery Activities**: To stay aware of motivation, select fun proactive assignments. This could consolidate moving, climbing, developing, or regardless, participating in sports like tennis or golf.

In the event that you've been lethargic for a long time or are new to working out, start cautiously. Consistently increase the power and term of your activities as you go.

- **Work it Up:** Use various activities to target different muscle social occasions and keep things new in your program. This could incorporate a mix of activities for balance, strength, versatility, and high-influence work out.

- **Hydrate**: Staying by and large around hydrated is basic for staying aware of general prosperity, especially for additional carefully prepared individuals.

- **Center around Your Body**: Give close thought to how your body feels while rehearsing and from that point. Develop your penchant or talk with a clinical consideration provider in the event that you cultivate torture or pain.

- Stay aware of Consistency: Practice appreciates many advantages, in any case, given that you dependably get it going. Meaning to do something like 150 minutes of moderate-force oxygen-consuming development or 75 minutes of energetic power enthusiastic activity every week, together with no less than two days of muscle-supporting work.

Consistently recollect that it's never beyond the place where it is feasible to start being dynamic and that there are many advantages to rehearsing for good development. To participate in a more cheerful, better, and more powerful developing endeavor, change your health routine to your unique essentials and capacities and spotlight it for the rest of your life.

B.Bodily-Cerebrum Affiliation

The cerebrum body interface, as it is in some cases alluded to, is the connection between an individual's psychological and actual well-being and thriving (body) and genuine prosperity and flourishing (mind). This association has been broadly contemplated and bantered across certain areas, including mind examination, medications, and thinking. Coming up next are huge components of the mind-body interface:

The body and mind are not viewed as being free elements by the cerebrum-body relationship, but rather as being interconnected and significantly affecting each other according to an expansive viewpoint. This perspective underlines the significance of considering both mental and real parts to grasp well-being and disease.

2. Psychosomatic Wellbeing: Psychosomatic illnesses happen when mental factors generally add to the acceleration, movement, or bother of real aftereffects. Pressure-related issues like Krabbe entrail condition and stressed cerebral throbs are remembered as psychosomatic problems.

3. Self-affected result: A self-impacted outcome is an eccentricity where a patient feels like their secondary effects or in general well-being have improved despite getting treatment that has no helpful advantage. This impact exhibits the impact of the mind on real prosperity results.

4. Stress and Feelings: Drawn out pressure, tension, weighty sentiments, and different circumstances that are private to an individual could affect their real prosperity. For example, long-stretch strain has been connected to some medical issues, including heart issues, circulatory issues, and stomach-related unsettling influences.

5. Mind-Body Meditations: A few remedial methodologies and prescriptions try to utilize the brain-body association with upgraded recuperation and prosperity. Yoga, caring pursuits, thoughtfulness, and unwinding procedures are completely integrated into the models. These strategies accentuate the benefit of keeping up with one's psychological and neighborhood prosperity to safeguard one's general prosperity.

6. Psychoneuroimmunology: This field of examination investigates the connections between the neurological, safe, and mental cycles. It investigates the effect of mental factors like feelings, pressure, and different elements on tough reactions and by and large prosperity.

7. Biofeedback: Individuals can screen and control explicit physiological cycles, like a heartbeat or strong tension, by utilizing non stop investigation. It very well may be utilized by individuals to bring down their pulse and upgrade their general well-being.

8. Mind-Body Medication: Mind-body medication is an all-encompassing way to deal with medical services that recognize the meaning of social, philosophical, and mental perspectives in one's genuine achievement. It intermittently consolidates standard strategies with equal medicines to work on by and large well-being.

9. Care-Based Tension Abatement (MBSR): MBSR is a deliberate methodology that consolidates care thought and yoga to assist individuals with overseeing pressure, diminishing the outcomes of various problems, and working on their pleasure.

10. Mind-Body Associations in Constant Ailment: In ongoing circumstances, the psyche-body association is especially significant. For contaminations like fibromyalgia, ongoing torment, and resistant framework sicknesses, a total way to deal with treatment is earnestly required because these circumstances often involve baffling collaborations among mental and genuine parts.

The probability of the cerebrum-body relationship underlines that it is critical to grasp how mental and actual prosperity are associated. Knowing how these two things are connected can assist us with growing smart medical care and flourishing methodologies that consider how our mentalities, convictions, and personal conduct standards influence our physical and profound prosperity.

I..How emotional well-being influences life span

Since an individual's emotional well-being can influence various pieces of their life, including those that ultimately influence their general prosperity and actual well-being, it can extensively affect how long they live. Here are a few different ways that emotional wellness might affect life span:

1. Actual Wellbeing: Issues with actual well-being can result from psychological well-being issues like delayed pressure, tension, and gloom. For example, steady pressure could expand an individual's gamble of creating coronary illness, hypertension, and other ongoing illnesses that can lessen life expectancy.

2. Wellbeing Propensities: Individuals with poor emotional well-being could be more inclined to undesirable propensities including smoking, hitting the bottle hard, eating inadequately, and not working out. These activities can abbreviate life expectancies and add to the development of some well-being issues.

3. Treatment Adherence: Individuals who fight with psychological well-being problems might find it challenging to follow recommended clinical medicines for actual ailments. They endanger getting more debilitated and carrying on with more limited lives if they don't consume their medications or treatments as recommended.

4. Social Disengagement: Emotional well-being issues can bring about depression and social detachment. The absence of social help and significant associations can seriously affect one's physical and psychological wellness, which can eventually abbreviate one's life expectancy.

5. Self-Care: Individuals who have solid emotional well-being are more disposed to embrace taking care of oneself exercises including getting ordinary activity, eating a sound eating regimen, and finding support from a specialist when essential. These schedules can uphold work on actual well-being and protect life.

6. Immunological Capability: Long-haul pressure and psychological wellness issues can disable immunological capability, leaving individuals more inclined to diseases and ailments. A debilitated safe framework might cause an abbreviated life expectancy.

7. Self-destruction Hazard: Serious emotional wellness that is left untreated can, in certain circumstances, bring about self-destruction, which is a significant worldwide reason for an early demise.

8. Personal satisfaction: Psychological well-being hardships may not be guaranteed to bring about actual medical problems, but rather they can in any case considerably affect an individual's overall personal satisfaction. Bad quality of life could diminish one's craving to live, which might in a roundabout way affect life span.

The connection between emotional well-being and life span is confounded and impacted by certain factors, including hereditary qualities, financial level, admittance to medical care, and the presence of social help. Early discovery and viable emotional wellness treatment can reduce the harmful impacts of these circumstances on actual wellbeing and upgrade general prosperity, which might assist with people carrying on with longer and better lives.

Ii. Care and stress decrease

You may decisively upgrade your psychological and profound prosperity by joining pressure decrease and care strategies. Together, they are habitually utilized to help individuals in beating hindrances in day to day existence and decrease the adverse outcomes of stress. Here is a synopsis of the two thoughts and instances of how they may be utilized:

1. Stress The executives: Stress the board is an assortment of strategies and thoughts planned to reduce the physiological, profound, and mental responses to stressors. Stress is a piece of life and is typical, however drawn out or unnecessary pressure can hurt your wellbeing and general personal satisfaction. You can recuperate control and harmony by rehearsing successful pressure on the board.

Techniques for Overseeing Pressure:

   a. Decide Stressors: To begin, pinpoint the exact wellsprings of your pressure. The causes could be natural, individual, or business related.

   b. Using time productively: Put forth boundaries for your errands and appropriately deal with your opportunity to decrease sensations of over-burden.

C. Solid Way of life: Customary activity, a reasonable eating routine, and sufficient rest are pivotal for overseeing pressure.

D. Unwinding Procedures: Drawn out profound breathing, continuous muscle unwinding, and contemplation can all help you loosen up and bring down your feelings of anxiety.

E. Social Help: Talk with friends and family about your concerns, or contemplate joining support gatherings.

f. Look for Proficient Help: In the event that your anxiety surpasses your ability to deal with it, you should talk with a specialist or guide for counsel and backing.

2. Mindfulness: Care is a psychological activity that includes zeroing in on the current second without judgment. It pushes you to recognize your sentiments, considerations, and body encounters without endeavoring to adjust them. Despite the fact that care is oftentimes connected to contemplation, it very well might be integrated into day to day existence in more ways than one.

Care strategies:

a. Care reflection involves sitting discreetly and focusing on your breath or some specific part of the ongoing second.

Cautious unwinding can be delivered simply by zeroing in on your inward breath and breathing out.

c. Play out a psychological body check, noticing any snugness or different sensations you might be feeling as you go from head to toe.

D. Cautious Eating: Take as much time as necessary and partake in each chomp, giving close consideration to the flavor, appearance, and fragrance of your food.

a. Walk carefully and gradually, focusing on how your body moves and the sensations in your feet.

The Connection Between Care and Stress Decrease:

Care can be a reasonable technique for focusing on the board since it builds your consciousness of your stressors and your reactions to them. Partaking in care practices will assist you with refining your strategy for practical adaptations and figuring out how to respond to pressure in a more made and imperturbable way. Care likewise empowers self-sympathy, which is useful for changing following pressure.

Coordinating strain decline techniques and care rehearses into your day-to-day schedule can bring about a more dynamic and peaceful presence. As you start your excursion toward stress decrease and more huge treatment, practice restraint. Recollect that fostering these abilities requires some investment, exertion, and practice.

C. Public permeability and local area inclusion

The expression "social and neighborhood" alludes to individuals, affiliations, and gatherings effectively captivating in drives and exercises intended to reinforce networks and the help of their constituents from the public authority. People team up to track down answers for issues, reinforce social ties, and impact positive change. Responsibility on a worldwide, social, and nearby level is fundamental for social orders to find success. Coming up next are a few fundamental parts of social and neighborhood responsibility:

1. Volunteering: One of the main types of neighborhood association is assisting. It involves individuals loaning their assets, abilities, and time to help different associations, missions, or causes. Volunteers are important in resolving social issues, offering principal types of assistance, and cultivating social ties.

2. Civil Responsibility: Civil responsibility envelop exercises like projecting a voting structure in choices, going to public occasions, and having political conversations. It gives people the opportunity to partake in choices that influence their organizations and countries.

3. Region neighborhood Arranging: Nearby facilitators unite people to team up on issues that both of them view as significant. They coordinate assets, have social gatherings, and make intentions to resolve specific issues or encourage tremendous change in a neighborhood.

4. Social Activism: Those who work for change in friendly, political, or natural issues are alluded to as well-disposed activists. They utilize various strategies, including presentations, petitions, and mindfulness crusades, to pass on data and request administrative changes.

5. Neighborhood: Endeavors to help a neighborhood thrive are viewed as neighborhood. This classification might incorporate ventures that give a structure, monetary result, instructive, clinical, and social help.

6. Framework organization and facilitated exertion: Coordinated effort between individuals, gatherings, associations, and state-run administrations is much of the time essential for organizations to be effectively attracted. Making and keeping up with gatherings and associations will empower the neighborhood to have a huge effect.

7. Instruction and Care: Illuminating individuals about unambiguous issues, like social liberties, generally speaking, prosperity, or ecological assurance, is a fundamental part of local area support. Schooling and information scattering can impact conduct and assist with settling on informed choices.

8. Variety and Inclusivity: A compelling social class responsibility ought to be wide, and welcoming to people of all foundations, ages, and capacities. To be versatile, networks should be areas of strength to have, which calls for embracing distinction and encouraging a feeling of having a place.

9. Social Capital: Alluded to as the social bonds, trust, and normal standards of a social class. It is fundamental for the goal of issues, the use of assets, and the overall thriving of occupants in the area.

10. Assessment and Info: For deciding the adequacy of neighborhood drives and making the fundamental changes, it is vital to watch and dissect them. Because of the neighborhood, tasks and activities are chipped away at.

Less disparity, a better life, and a firm labor force are only a couple of the drawn-out benefits of social and neighborhood local contribution. It enables individuals to contribute to guaranteeing a superior future for their organizations and themselves.

I. The meaning of associations with others

Social connections play an essential part in our lives since they enormously upgrade our general joy and joy. The significance of social ties is exhibited by the rundown of components below:

1. Daily reassurance: Social ties offer an organization of companions, family members, and friends who can be a wellspring of help while confronting tough spots. Stress, tension, and bitterness can be decreased by conversing with individuals about your viewpoints and sentiments.

Solid social bonds have been connected to better actual well-being, as indicated by certain examinations. Solid social ties are related to longer life expectancies, diminished rate of ongoing illnesses, and speedier recuperation from affliction.

Social ties are fundamental for keeping up with solid emotional well-being, which carries us to number three. The probability of emotional well-being conditions including sadness and social tension is diminished by friendly association and helps fight depression. It provides one with a sensation of motivation and having a place.

4. Decrease of Pressure: Social encouraging groups of people can act as a pressure minimizer. It very well may be more straightforward to deal with testing conditions when you realize you have people you can depend on. It can likewise be great and quiet to have discussions and offer encounters with buddies.

5. Self-improvement: Collaborating with a shifted scope of people opens you to different perspectives and contemplations. Thus, one might encounter self-improvement, more noteworthy compassion, and a more extensive point of view on the world.

6. Contentment: A major figure of joy and life fulfillment is social ties. Carrying on with a brighter life includes getting things done with loved ones, commending achievements, and gaining inestimable experiences.

7. Systems administration and Possibilities: Social connections can offer ways to open doors in both individual and expert life. For example, organizing with individuals in your field might bring about employment opportunities or cooperative ventures. Special interactions could bring about intriguing experiences and undertakings.

8. Resilience: Individuals who have solid informal organizations have an emotionally supportive network that permits them to recuperate all the more rapidly from difficulties. Loved ones can urge individuals to defeat snags, whether it accompanies a material guide or daily encouragement.

9. Feeling of Having a Place: Social ties assist people in feeling like they have a place and are what their identity is. The reason for an individual's character can be laid by feeling a piece of a local area or gathering.

10. Longevity: Concentrates routinely show that those with solid social ties will quite often live longer. A superior and seriously fulfilling life can be worked with by the psychological and actual help that these organizations give.

Our prosperity and self-improvement rely upon social connections, which are not only a pleasant component of life. A principal part of carrying on with a blissful and satisfying life is

developing and encouraging these associations.
Our associations with others — whether they
accompany family, companions, or our networks
— hugely affect how blissful we are all in all.

Ii. Making senior-accommodating areas

For seniors' general prosperity and personal
satisfaction, making steady communities is
fundamental. These areas look to provide senior
residents with a feeling of the local area,
admittance to vital administrations, and
opportunities for social cooperation. Here are
significant cycles and things to ponder while
growing such networks:

1. Needs Evaluation: To start, embrace a
careful requirements examination to discover the
specific necessities and inclinations of the senior

populace in your space. Reviews, center gatherings, and conversations with senior consideration and gerontology experts might be essential for this interaction.

2. Open Lodging: Guarantee that the scope of lodging decisions is offered, including open and reasonable lodging. To oblige those with portability issues, contemplate consolidating highlights like snatch bars, more extensive passageways, and inclines while building new homes or redesigning existing ones.

3. Medical care Administrations: Cooperate with medical care providers to follow through on-location medical care and health administrations. This can include normal exams, actual therapy, advising for psychological wellness issues, and help to oversee ongoing illnesses.

4. Transportation: Set up open and reasonable transportation decisions, for example, transport administrations or joint efforts with provincial transportation organizations, to make it simpler for more seasoned residents to move around the area and access vital administrations.

5. Get-togethers: Make a schedule of social events that are fit for seniors' inclinations and limits. These could incorporate studios for expressions and artworks, writing clubs, cultivating gatherings, and trips to local widespread developments.

6. Chipping in Valuable open doors: Advance intergenerational connections by allowing senior residents to chip in and give their experience and aptitude to more youthful ages. This advances a sensation of association and reason.

7. Public venues: Make people group centers or regions for social events where elderly folks can gather, blend, and take part in a scope of exercises. Support gatherings and informative talks can likewise be held at these offices.

8. Care Coordination: Offer consideration coordination administrations to more seasoned residents to help them explore the medical services framework, acquire benefits, and layout associations with neighborhood assets and care groups.

9. Wellbeing and Security: To guarantee occupant well-being, put crisis reaction frameworks, nonstop security, and standard wellbeing reviews set up.

10. Innovation Combination: Incorporate mechanical arrangements that can work on the existences of old residents, for example, telemedicine administrations, shrewd home mechanization to assist with regular errands, and advanced specialized devices to stay in contact with companions.

11. Social Responsiveness: Be comprehensive and delicate to different societies to address the issues of seniors who come from various foundations. Offering food, diversion, and backing administrations that are appropriate for the way of life is important for this.

12. Local area Inclusion: Remember more established residents for dynamic cycles and rouse them to effectively take part in shaping the local area. Upgrades and a more noteworthy feeling of pride might result from their commitment.

13. Partnerships: Cooperate with local organizations, legislative establishments, and not-for-profits that offer senior administrations to pool assets and skills.

14. Training and Mindfulness: Run outreach and instructive exercises to get the message out about more established residents' necessities and the assets that are presented in the area.

15. Reliable information: Gather input from seniors and their families to persistently assess the adequacy of the local area's administrations and make required adjustments.

It takes cautious preparation, consistent commitment, and a multidisciplinary way to deal with making senior-accommodating networks. You can make an exuberant, inviting climate where older folks can progress in years with respect and a great life by taking care of their physical, profound, social, and medical services prerequisites.

D. Tweaked Long-haul Plans

Customized answers for a more drawn out, better life are known as customized life span plans. These plans offer guidance and directions for expanding an individual's life and further developing their prosperity by thinking about their specific hereditary qualities, way of life, and clinical history. Coming up next are a few fundamental components of a remarkable lifespan plan:

1. Wellbeing Assessment: Begin by deciding your present status of well-being. This can involve intensive clinical assessments, for example, blood tests, hereditary testing, and expert clinical guidance.

2. Alterations to your lifestyle include: - Diet: Change your eating regimen to meet your wholesome necessities while considering your sensitivities, awarenesses, and inherited inclinations. A decent, supplement-thick eating routine high in organic products, vegetables, entire grains, lean meats, and solid fats ought to be the principal center.

- **exercise**: Make a modified exercise plan that considers your ongoing degree of wellness, your targets, and any actual limitations. Incorporate exercises for both strength preparation and heart-stimulating exercises.

- **Stress the executives**: Incorporate pressure-decrease rehearses like yoga, contemplation, or care in your day-to-day practice to reduce the adverse results of progressing pressure.

- **Sleep**: Give quality rest a need by giving a loosening up dozing climate and a standard rest routine.

- **Stay away from Negative ways of behaving:** Perceive and dispose of awful ways of behaving including smoking, hard-core boozing, and medication utilization.

3. Hereditary Experiences: Utilize hereditary testing to get familiar with your hereditary defenselessness to explicit clinical issues. Individualized safeguard plans and early gamble distinguishing proof can be directed by this information.

4. Preventive Medical care: Stay up to date with proposed tests and vaccinations. Cooperate with your PCP to treat any continuous issues or other medical problems immediately.

5. Dietary Enhancements: Think about including supplements, like nutrients, minerals, or different supplements, in your eating routine because of your specific requests and dietary deficiencies.

6. Center around mental and profound prosperity by participating in exercises that encourage close-to-home prosperity, like normal social cooperation, leisure activities, and directing when essential, and by putting psychological wellness first.

7. Social Associations: Encourage strong connections and keep a functioning social schedule. Social connections might be connected to life span, as indicated by research.

8. Mental Wellbeing: Remain intellectually fit by taking part in deep-rooted learning and mental exercises. Participate in practices that test your mental capacity.

9. Plan Ordinary Well Being Tests: To follow your prosperity and alter your life span methodology as the need might arise, plan routine well-being assessments and screenings.

10. Remain Informed: Stay aware of the latest examinations on life span, maturing, and wellbeing. Your individualized methodology could change because of late logical revelations.

11. Flexibility: Know that when your objectives, targets, and conditions change over the long run, your life span plan may likewise require changes.

12. Monetary Preparation: Guarantee that your life span system incorporates monetary wanting to guarantee that you have the assets to help a more extended life.

Recollect that individualized life span plans ought to be made related to clinical experts who can offer proficient heading and observing. Making the procedure explicitly for your necessities and circumstances is essential since what works for one individual may not be proper for another.

I..Tailoring strategies for determined requirements and goals

The capacity to adjust procedures to meet exceptional prerequisites and targets is vital for both individual and expert turn of events. Changing your methodology can drastically build your possibilities of succeeding, whether or not your objectives are proficient achievement, mindfulness, or accomplishment in one more aspect of your life. Consider the accompanying activities while changing your arrangements to unequivocal prerequisites and targets:

1. Self-Reflection; To begin, assess your benefits and downsides, proclivities, and values. What are your forthcoming and critical objectives? Which spikes would you say you are riding? What principles do you have? Care is the most important phase in creating one of a kind systems.

2. Obviously Express Your Objectives: Obviously express your objectives in a manner that is quantitative, reachable, huge, and time-bound (Splendid). Creating techniques to help explicit points is more straightforward.

3. Assess Your Resources: Become mindful of the devices you have available to you. Your abilities, data, available energy, resources that are effectively open, and accomplice association are totally remembered for this. Realizing your resources will assist you with making astonishing game plans.

4. Focus on Your Objectives: Assuming that you have a few objectives, request them as indicated by significance and need. Focus on one or a couple of essential objectives immediately to try not to allow yourself to go to pieces.

5. Make movement plans that are intended for every objective. Stage five is this. Decide the exact undertakings, occupations, and finish times important to meet your objectives. These strategies should be adaptable and responsive to changes or disasters.

6.Zeroing in on fostering your aptitudes can assist you with affecting your resources. Utilize your assets for your potential benefit to accomplish your objectives. This might build your motivation and certainty.

7. Right Deformities: Perceive your inadequacies and where you can move along. Plan ways of tending to or conquer these inadequacies, for example, by acquiring new abilities or requesting help.

8. Agree with Learning Styles: While securing new information or abilities, consider your favored learning strategy. Perusing, taking part in learning, and utilizing visual guides are powerful learning strategies. Change your appearance processes as the need might arise.

9. Dealing with your time well: Make your time usage procedures fit your regular schedules and propensities. Which do you really want, morning or night? Work on over longer or more limited periods?

10. Request Ideas: Be open to ideas from trusted specialists, colleagues, or coaches. They could give accommodating direction and help you in changing your strategies on a case by case basis.

11. Be versatile: Since life is strange, anything could occur. Continuously concoct an alternate arrangement when it is proper. Flexibility is fundamental for handling new difficulties and potential results.

12. Follow Your Advancement: Continually assess how far you've come. Do you have an agreement? Is it true or not that you are fruitful in arriving at your objectives?
Make any fundamental changes utilizing this analysis.

13. Observe Victories: Commend every one of your humble triumphs en route. Perceiving your triumphs can help your inspiration and keep you zeroed in on your goals.

14. Be Dependable: It requires investment to change a method to meet an individual's prerequisites and objectives. Obligation and dependability are essential for a relentless cycle. Keep up with your technique improvement as you push ahead.

15. Request Help: Go ahead and move toward tutors, care gatherings, or guides for help. On the way, they can give you direction, obligation, and backing.

Always remember that fostering a technique to suit an individual's necessities and objectives is a close to home and iterative cycle. Since what works for one individual probably won't work for another, it is critical to overhaul your framework to represent your special circumstances and objectives.

Ii. The job of clinical specialists in giving individualized treatment

To furnish patients with individualized care, medical services specialists are fundamental. Customized care, some of the time alluded to as customized medication or accuracy medication, is a strategy that changes a patient's clinical consideration and medical care decisions to their novel clinical requirements. To make the most proficient and individualized therapy plan, this strategy thinks about a patient's specific hereditary cosmetics, way of life, inclinations, and clinical history. Parts of the job of medical services experts in giving individualized care incorporate the accompanying:

1. Evaluation and Conclusion: Medical services suppliers are responsible for aggregating complete information on the patient's hereditary cosmetics, clinical history, and family and social history. They utilize this information to precisely analyze the patient's sickness and to see as any unmistakable hereditary or biomarker-based attributes that could have an effect.

2. Genomic medication: In specific conditions, medical services experts might utilize genomic information to all the more likely comprehend a patient's gamble factors or pick the most reasonable course of treatment. Deciphering hereditary information and depicting its ramifications to patients is habitually finished by hereditary instructors and geneticists.

3. Treatment Arranging: Cooperating, medical care experts make a particular therapy plan for every patient considering their unmistakable profile. Contingent upon the patient's requests and hereditary attributes, this technique might include prescription choice, portions, and treatment lengths that are altered.

4. Observing and Change: Customized care requires progressing evaluation of the patient's turn of events and any conceivable adverse consequences. To work on the patient's well being and prosperity, medical care specialists assess therapy results routinely and change as needs be.

5. Shared Direction: Customized care puts areas of strength for an on correspondence and agreement working among patients and medical services experts. Experts prompt patients about accessible medicines, potential dangers, and benefits, engaging them to settle on choices that are in accordance with their qualities and inclinations.

6. Patient Schooling: Medical services suppliers are accountable for illuminating patients about their illnesses, accessible therapies, and way of life changes. They give ideas on how individuals can play a functioning job in their consideration and really deal with their wellbeing.

7. Coordination of Care: In complex cases, a few medical services suppliers, for example, essential consideration specialists, trained professionals, attendants, and drug specialists, might be participating in a patient's consideration. To ensure that the patient gets individualized and intensive consideration, viable correspondence and coordination between these suppliers is significant.

8. Moral Contemplations: Medical services specialists should oversee moral issues connected with individualized care, like safeguarding patient protection, getting educated assent for hereditary testing, and managing any possible disgrace or segregation connected to hereditary data.

9. Innovative work: Medical care experts likewise help to advance redid medication by doing research and staying up to date with the latest headways in the field. They could partake in clinical preliminaries, add to the assortment of clinical information, and adjust new operations and advancements into their standard practices.

10. Proceeding with Training: Since the field of customized medication is growing rapidly, medical care experts should keep on figuring out how to keep awake to date with the most current indicative procedures, treatments, and proposals.

All in all, medical care experts have a vital impact in giving individualized care by changing therapy plans and clinical decisions following the exceptional patient highlights. The personal satisfaction for people getting customized care can be expanded because of this procedure, which can likewise bring about more viable and proficient medical services.

Chapter 4

Different Considerations on Physician recommended Medications for Life Span

Different contemplations of "Medication forever" include moving the focal point of clinical benefits from exclusively restoring ailments to quickly expanding and dragging out solid life expectancies. This technique incorporates various strategies and convictions that plan to build individuals' satisfaction and the quantity of solid, useful years they appreciate as they age. While contemplating long-haul medication, remember the accompanying significant focuses:

1. Preventive Drug: Stress counteraction procedures incorporate antibodies, dietary changes, and early screenings to recognize and treat medical problems before they decline.

2. Modified Prescription: Tailor clinical medicines and medications to an individual's acquired qualities, lifestyle, and explicit well-being prerequisites.

3. Individual style Reflections: - Energize sound way of life decisions like standard activity, adjusted nourishment, stress the board, and satisfactory rest because these perspectives immensely affect the future.

4. Medicines Went Against Precise Maturing: Research in areas including regenerative medication, epigenetics, and senescence tries to foster treatments that defer the framework's maturing at the phone and subatomic levels.

5. Exactness Drug: Utilize current diagnostics and biomarker observation to distinguish disease risk factors early, considering designated medications and treatments.

6. Telemedicine and Remote Checking: - Use development to give clinical consideration benefits from good ways, check for tireless sicknesses, and give speedy clinical exhortation, particularly for the elderly and those with restricted versatility.

7. Healthspan versus life length: Centers around expanding prosperity range, or how much time that people are sound areas of strength for and, went against just broadening life expectancy.

8. Geriatric prescription: - Think about the older populace's extraordinary clinical necessities and difficulties while creating models and clinical consideration frameworks.

9. Life-length investigation: Put subsidies in research that ganders at the fundamental models for developing to help medications that can defer or change the developing framework.

10. Social Determinants of Prosperity: - Address social and monetary factors that influence prosperity and admittance to clinical treatment, as these can significantly affect the future.

11. Lead Monetary Angles: Apply social monetary standards to encourage more noteworthy judgment and consistency with remedial guidance.

12. Moral Considerations: Consider moral problems connected with life span, like admittance to state-of-the-art drugs, fair admittance to clinical treatment, and living a "fantastic" or "fulfilled" life in advanced age.

13. Technique and Rule: Adjust clinical consideration procedures and suggestions to help life-length-focused requests, progressions, and drives.

14. Public Care: Illuminate the overall population about the advantages of a proactive way to deal with maturing as well as the requirement for life-length focused clinical consideration.

It requires collaboration from clinical experts, specialists, officials, and the overall local area to address the different contemplations encompassing prescription for life term. A sweeping way to deal with medical services expects to enable people to assume responsibility for their well-being and work on their thriving all through their lives.

A.Moving from Illness Treatment to Avoidance

The progress from sickness therapy to illness counteraction is a fundamental thought in medical services that has filled in importance lately. This change shows a proactive procedure for saving and further developing general well-being as opposed to just responding to disease when it emerges. This shift is basic because of multiple factors:

1. Cost-Effectiveness: Sickness avoidance is habitually more practical than infection therapy. Treating constant sicknesses and dealing with the repercussions of preventable infections can be expensive and overburden medical care frameworks. Medical care assets can be better used by putting resources into counteraction.

2. Expanded Personal satisfaction:
Anticipation centers around keeping people solid and bringing down their opportunity of infection. People's satisfaction improves as they stay away from the aggravation and limits related to different infections.

3. Decreased Medical services disparities:
Counteraction exercises can help with reducing medical care imbalances by focusing on weak populations and giving admittance to protection administrations. This might bring about more pleasant medical service results.

4. Long-haul Well-being: Preventive intercessions regularly help long-haul wellbeing and prosperity. Sound practices, like ordinary activity, adjusted nourishment, and stress the board, can assist with keeping away from a wide range of ongoing illnesses.

5. Decreased disease Weight: Powerful ailment preventive measures can decrease the general weight of infections in society. This envelops actual well-being as well as the close-to-home and monetary cost that sicknesses take on people and society.

Here are a few critical strategies for changing toward disease counteraction:

1. Wellbeing Instruction: Raise public mindfulness and instruction about sound ways of life, risk factors, and the meaning of normal check-ups and antibodies.

2. Inoculation Projects: Support and extend immunization projects to forestall irresistible illnesses and slow their spread.

3. Screening and Early Identification: Urge standard well-being tests to find infections at a prior, more treatable stage. Mammograms, colonoscopies, and pulse checks are a couple of models.

4. Way of life Intercessions: To limit the gamble of ongoing illnesses, advance solid ways of behaving like normal active work, a decent eating regimen, smoking discontinuance, and stress the executives.

5. Natural and Strategy enhancements: Advocate for regulation and natural enhancements that advance better networks, like expanding admittance to quality food varieties, lessening air contamination, and making safe regions for active work.

6. Medical services Framework Accentuation: Urge medical services professionals to zero in on anticipation through routine screenings, preventive consideration meetings, and patient training.

7. Social Financial matters: Utilize social financial matters standards to make medicines that urge individuals to go with better decisions.

8. Exploration and Development: Put resources into exploration to recognize new preventive measures and innovations.

9. Public-Private Organizations: Team up with private area gatherings, non-benefits, and state-run administrations to lay out extensive precaution programs.

Generally, changing from disease treatment to counteraction requires a diverse methodology including people, medical services suppliers, states, and the bigger society. It is an interest in the drawn-out well-being and prosperity of people and society in general, with the possibility of bringing down medical care costs and working on by and large personal satisfaction.

I . The idea of preventive medication

Deterrent medication, otherwise called preventive medication or preventive medical care, is a clinical practice that spotlights keeping up with and improving general well-being and prosperity by forestalling the development of sicknesses, mishaps, or other well-being problems before they emerge or deteriorate. This part of medication underscores the need to make preventive moves to decrease the weight of the disorder and advance a better populace. Here are a few vital standards of precaution medication:

1. Wellbeing Advancement and Instruction: Protection medication regularly incorporates general well-being efforts, instructive drives, and individual guidance to bring issues to light about sound ways of life, risk factors, and the requirement for early location and intercession.

2. Vaccinations: Vaccinations are a significant part of safeguard medication. Immunizations assist with shielding people and society from irresistible sicknesses by initiating the resistant framework to produce insusceptibility against explicit contaminations.

3. Way of life Alteration: Empowering people to take on better propensities like eating a decent eating routine, participating in customary actual work, stopping smoking, and restricting liquor utilization can essentially diminish Constant issues like coronary illness, diabetes, and a few malignancies in danger.

4. Screening and Early Location: Precaution medication accentuates customary screenings and check-ups to reveal well-being problems in their beginning phases. Mammograms for bosom disease, colonoscopies for colorectal malignant growth, and pulse checks for hypertension are a couple of models.

5. Hereditary Guiding: On the off chance that an individual has a family background of hereditary irregularities or is in danger of acquiring specific circumstances, hereditary directing can give data and assist on how to deal with these dangers.

6. Ecological Wellbeing: One more piece of preventive medication is distinguishing and moderating natural factors that can affect well-being. This incorporates handling issues like air and water contamination, working environment risks, and poison openness.

7. Prescription and Treatment: Some precautionary medication strategies incorporate the utilization of drugs or treatments to limit the gamble of explicit illnesses. Statins, for instance, might be prescribed to bring down cholesterol levels and limit the gamble of coronary illness.

8. Medical Care Strategy and General Wellbeing Drives: States and medical services associations assume a significant part in preventive medication by creating arrangements and projects pointed toward advancing general well-being. These may incorporate food naming guidelines, cigarette control endeavors, and subsidizing for research on preventive measures.

9. Individualized Medication: Propels in hereditary qualities and innovation have empowered the advancement of individualized precaution mediations in light of a person's hereditary structure and special well-being risk factors.

Safeguarding medication is basic to bringing down medical services costs, working on personal satisfaction, and expanding the absolute future. This procedure attempts to move the focal point of medical services from essentially treating diseases toward effectively saving well-being and prosperity by focusing on anticipation and early intercession. An interdisciplinary region unites medical care suppliers, general well-being specialists, policymakers, and people to advance better living and lower sickness trouble.

Ii. Coordinating genomes and chance evaluation

Coordinating hereditary qualities into risk evaluation is a new and quickly growing subject that can possibly change how we might interpret redid wellbeing gambles and illuminate custom-made medical services intercessions. Here are a few significant qualities of combining genomes and hazard evaluation:

1. **Hereditary Gamble Elements:** Genomic information can give critical data about a person's hereditary inclination to different infections. Specialists and medical care professionals can find explicit hereditary variations connected to an expanded gamble of illnesses like malignant growth, coronary illness, diabetes, and others by assessing a person's hereditary piece.

2. **Polygenic Gamble Scores (PRS):** Polygenic gamble scores are resolved in light of the total

impact of a few hereditary varieties related to a specific illness. These scores give a more thorough evaluation of a person's hereditary gamble for a specific condition. PRS can be utilized to order people and guide individualized preventive and screening programs.

3. Individual Hereditary Guiding and Instruction: Incorporating genomics into risk appraisal requires able hereditary guiding and schooling for people. Patients should comprehend their hereditary gamble factors, the restrictions of hereditary testing, and the ramifications of their outcomes. Hereditary advisors assume a significant part in empowering these discourses.

4. Clinical Choice Help: Medical care experts can utilize genomic information to illuminate clinical direction. A patient with a high innate gamble for bosom malignant growth, for instance, might be urged to start mammography screening at a prior age or to investigate risk-diminishing measures like preventive medical procedure or medicine.

5. Pharmacogenomics: Genomic information can likewise be used to redo pharmacological treatment plans. Pharmacogenomics looks at a person's hereditary varieties to guess how they will respond to explicit medications. This can assist with further developing medication choice and portion to boost helpful advantages while lessening adverse consequences.

6. Way of life Change: Incorporating hereditary qualities into risk evaluation can empower people to pursue informed way of life decisions. For instance, in the event that somebody has a hereditary penchant to weight, they might get individualized sustenance and exercise ideas to diminish their gamble.

7. Exploration and Disclosure: Coordinating genomic information can support the disclosure of novel hereditary gamble elements and infection pathways. This information might prompt the improvement of new drugs and medications.

8. Moral and Protection Concerns: As genomics turns out to be more coordinated into risk appraisal and treatment, it is basic to address moral and security concerns. Guaranteeing the classification and security of genomic information is basic, as is acquiring informed assent from the people who attempt hereditary testing.

9. Information Mix: To give a careful gamble evaluation, genomic information ought to be joined with other clinical and natural variables. This envelops things like family ancestry, way of life, and ecological openings.

10. Cost and Openness: To guarantee fair access for all populaces, more noteworthy coordination of genomics into risk appraisal ought to incorporate the expense adequacy and availability of hereditary testing and advising administrations.

All in all, integrating hereditary qualities into risk evaluation has critical commitment for further developing medical care by offering more custom-made and designated mediations. Nonetheless, it additionally presents issues concerning information insurance, moral contemplations, and medical services availability, which must all be painstakingly tended to as the area advances., which must all be painstakingly tended to as the area advances.

B.Targeting Maturing Itself

"Focusing on Maturing Itself" alludes to the idea of creating clinical medications and treatments that straightforwardly address the natural cycles of maturing, to expand human lifetime and lessen the weight of old enough related messes. This methodology is known as "maturing exploration" or "gerontology," and it mirrors a change away from treating individual sicknesses of maturing (like coronary illness, malignant growth, and dementia) and toward handling the central reasons for maturing itself.

The hypothesis behind focusing on maturing is that by contemplating and mediating in the major natural systems that drive maturing, researchers might have the option to forestall or try and converse a portion of the maturing related harm and decay that occurs in the human body over the long haul. Scientists are especially inspired by the accompanying maturing side effects:

1. Genomic Flimsiness: The amassing of DNA harm after some time.

2. Telomere Shortening: The progressive shortening of defensive covers on the closures of chromosomes.

3. Epigenetic Changes: Changes in quality articulation designs.

4. Loss of Proteostasis: A lessening in the body's capacity to keep up with protein capability.

5. Mitochondrial Brokenness: Decreased energy creation in cells.

6. Cell Senescence: The gathering of non-isolating, matured cells.

7. Undifferentiated cell Fatigue: Diminished recovery limit.

Changes in motioning between cells.

Analysts in this discipline are investigating various strategies and mediations to address these maturing side effects. These strategies might include the advancement of drugs or treatments that can fix DNA harm, reestablish telomere length, reset epigenetic marks, increment mitochondrial capability, take out senescent cells, or improve immature microorganism action.

Dr. Aubrey de Dark and the SENS Exploration Establishment, for instance, have lobbied for a comprehensive way to deal with maturing research known as "Systems for Designed Insignificant Senescence" (SENS). SENS proposes a blend of treatments to fix and recharge the body's tissues and frameworks, with a definitive objective of expanding a solid human lifetime.

While the subject of anti-maturing research is promising, numerous medications and treatments are still in the exploratory stage. Moral, administrative, and security contemplations are likewise significant in advancing these thoughts. Besides, it is urgent to note that maturing is a perplexing cycle, and creating a powerful enemy of maturing treatment might require a lot more long periods of exploration and testing.

I..The meaning of geroprotectors in expanding a solid life expectancy

Geroprotectors are synthetic compounds or treatments that can build a sound life expectancy by focusing on the basic components of maturing and age-related diseases. Expanding a sound life expectancy is an objective that has gotten a great deal of interest in the areas of gerontology and life span research. Here is a synopsis of the job of geroprotectors in this specific situation:

1. Deferring the beginning Old enough Related Illnesses: Geroprotectors attempt to defer or forestall the beginning Old enough related illnesses like coronary illness, disease, diabetes, Alzheimer's, and others. Thus, they can help people keep up with great well-being for a more drawn-out period, subsequently broadening the solid part of their lives.

2. Focusing on Maturing Trademarks: Specialists have distinguished different maturing trademarks, which are fundamental cycles or instruments that add to the maturing system. Geroprotectors are planned to address these trademarks, which might incorporate cell senescence, genomic insecurity, epigenetic changes, and mitochondrial disappointment.

3. Working on Cell Flexibility: A geroprotector's capability by working on the body's capacity to persevere through pressure and harm at the cell level. This can incorporate supporting DNA fix instruments, bringing down oxidative pressure, or expanding the freedom of harmed cells through cycles, for example, autophagy.

4. Caloric Limitation Mimetics: Caloric limitation (cutting calorie consumption without hunger) has been shown to increment life expectancy and further develop well-being in different animals. Caloric limitation mimetics are geroprotectors that attempt to copy the positive advantages of caloric limitation without the necessity for serious dietary regimens.

5. Senolytics: Senescence is what is happening in which cells lose their capacity to multiply and work ordinarily. Senescent cells can create maturing and lead to tissue breakdown and aggravation. Senolytics are geroprotectors that specifically annihilate senescent cells, possibly recovering tissues and upgrading general well-being.

6. Metabolic Intercessions: Some geroprotectors target metabolic pathways connected with maturing, like mTOR (mammalian objective of rapamycin) and AMPK (adenosine monophosphate-enacted protein kinase). Tweaking these pathways might well affect maturing-related processes.

7. Mitigating Impacts: Constant irritation is a run-of-the-mill part of maturing and age-related messes. Geroprotectors having mitigating exercises can assist with limiting the impending impacts of irritation and advance better maturing.

8. Way of life and Conduct Intercessions: While numerous geroprotectors are synthetic compounds or meds, way of life factors including normal activity, a reasonable eating regimen, and legitimate rest all assume a significant part in keeping a solid life expectancy. At the point when these activities are drilled reliably, they can be named geroprotective procedures.

9. Customized Approaches: It means quite a bit to take note that the viability of geroprotectors changes between people because of hereditary and natural elements. Customized ways to deal with geroprotector use, custom-made to a singular's particular well-being and hereditary profile, may turn out to be more applicable later on.

10. Moral and Wellbeing Issues: The utilization of geroprotectors presents moral and security issues, especially as they become all the more broadly accessible. Long-haul well-being studies and moral rules are expected to ensure that these medications are utilized morally and to serve people's well-being.

Geroprotectors show the possibility of broadening a sound life expectancy by tending to the fundamental reasons for maturing and age-related illnesses. While research in this area is continuous, the turn of events and appropriate use of geroprotective strategies can emphatically work on individuals' satisfaction as they age.

Ii. Clinical inceptions and imminent medicines.

Clinical fundamental examinations are comprehensive examinations done on human subjects to assess the security and adequacy of fresh out-of-plastic new clinical prescriptions, treatments, substances, headways, or mediations. These starter steps play a major part in the time spent making clinical benefits and making creative cures and drugs accessible for buying by the overall population. Here is a rundown of arranged treatments and clinical starter steps:

Clinical exploration for the most part advances through four stages:

1. Clinical Primer Stages

- In the primer stages, a specific number of solid workers or patients are utilized to explore the well-being and viability of a cunning remedy. The essential obligation is to settle on choices concerning the organization of the medicine and any possible adverse consequences.

Phase 2: In this step, a bigger gathering of patients gets the treatment to assess their overall well-being and practicality. The specialists should track down the ideal measurements and gather more data on possible antagonistic impacts.

- Phase 3: Primers for Stage 3 incorporate a bigger and more different gathering of patients to affirm the treatment's possibility, assess any adverse consequences, and contrast it with presently accessible standard prescriptions. The regulatory support requires specific major starter steps.

- Phase 4: Following regulatory freedom, Stage 4 primer evaluations (post-exhibiting perception) keep on looking at the treatment's drawn-out well-being and suitability in an unquestionable circumstance.

2. Clinical Primer Sorts: Clinical starter examination can zero in on various parts of clinical consideration, like medication improvement, clinical hardware, careful cycles, directing medicines, and the rundown continues forever. A few models are:

- Randomized Controlled Preliminaries (RCTs): Members are with no obvious end goal in mind relegated to treatment or control gatherings to concentrate on the impacts of another treatment, a fake treatment, or a current treatment.

- Observational Starters: These starter studies notice members in their regular surroundings without meddling or giving out medicine to find out about long-haul results.

- Crossbreed Starters: To look at individual responses, colleagues switch between various meds all through the request.

3. Anticipated drugs and Divulgences: Clinical fundamental examinations play had a basic impact in the improvement of various drugs and clinical forward leaps. The following are a couple of instances of models:

- Drugs: Clinical fundamentals are expected for assessing and demonstrating the viability of novel prescriptions for a scope of sicknesses, from vaccinations to threatening development treatments.

- Clinical Contraptions: Starters help decide the well-being and appropriateness of new clinical gadgets like prostheses, pacemakers, and suggestive gear.

- Excellent Treatments: CRISPR-based approaches and other great remedial examinations have created potential medicines for hereditary illnesses.

- Immunotherapies: Immunotherapy fundamental examination has shown an assurance in restoring specific diseases by utilizing the body's protected system to target harmful development cells.

- Exactness in Medication: Propels in genetic characteristics and further developed medicine have prompted the advancement of tweaked meds in light of a person's genetic profile.

- Social Medicines: Clinical primer examinations likewise inspect the possibility of considering diseases connected to an individual's propensities, close-to-home health, and lifestyle.

4. Authoritative Underwriting: Promising primer clinical outcomes are expected for managerial associations like the FDA (U.S. Food and Medicine Association) to embrace new prescriptions for boundless use.

5. Moral Reflections: Overseeing clinical preliminaries involves guaranteeing the ethical treatment of members, including acquiring informed assent and guarding their freedoms and security.

Clinical primers act as the establishment for clinical assessment, which thus moves the turn of events and endorsement of creative mediations, solutions, and treatments. Before these drugs are made generally accessible, they give the fundamental proof to lay out their adequacy and security.

C. The Significance of Interdisciplinary Joint Effort

The interdisciplinary joint effort is the course of experts from a few callings cooperating to resolve muddled issues, produce new arrangements, and advance information in manners that would be troublesome or difficult to do inside the constraints of a solitary discipline. This technique is getting some decent forward momentum and significance in different disciplines, including science, medical care, innovation, business, and the scholarly community. The following are a couple of motivations behind why interdisciplinary cooperation is basic:

1. All-encompassing Critical thinking:
Interdisciplinary groups can tackle complex issues by uniting fluctuated perspectives and ranges of abilities. This all-encompassing methodology considers a piece of full information on muddled issues, prompting more successful arrangements. Tending to environmental change, for instance, requires the contribution of researchers, architects, lawmakers, and financial analysts.

2. Inventiveness and Development: Cross-disciplinary joint effort advances inventiveness and development. At the point when individuals with assorted encounters and skills get together, they can give groundbreaking thoughts and viewpoints that can prompt forward leaps and extraordinary techniques. Developments, for example, the cell phone, which blends innovations from different disciplines, show the force of interdisciplinary ideas.

3. Better Direction: Interdisciplinary cooperation regularly prompts more educated navigation. At the point when experts from different callings work together, they might survey information according to numerous viewpoints and think about a more extensive scope of contemplations, bringing about additional balanced decisions. In medical services, for instance, a group of specialists, medical attendants, therapists, and social laborers can give more extensive patient consideration.

4. Tending to Complex Difficulties: Large numbers of the present most difficult issues are inherently interdisciplinary. Worldwide wellbeing pandemics, natural maintainability, and metropolitan arranging all require the interest of experts from different fields. Interdisciplinary cooperation accommodates a more planned and compelling reaction to these perplexing circumstances.

5. data Coordination: Interdisciplinary joint effort advances the mix of data from numerous spaces, prompting the improvement of new hypotheses, models, and approaches. This mix can help with beating holes across various fields and add to the development of human comprehension.

6. Further developing Instruction:
Interdisciplinary joint effort can likewise further develop instruction by presenting understudies to a more noteworthy scope of thoughts and methods. Interdisciplinary learning in training can all the more likely plan understudies for genuine circumstances and construct decisive abilities to reason.

7. Expanded Financing Amazing open doors:
Subsidizing offices and associations are progressively focusing on transdisciplinary examinations and drives. Cooperative endeavors often enjoy a cutthroat benefit concerning winning financing and assets since they are seen as bound to create significant outcomes.

8. Genuine Pertinence: In various ventures, similar to business and medical services, people are often compelled to work in interdisciplinary groups in reality. Interdisciplinary cooperation in schooling and research can plan people for these issues, making them more aggressive in the gig market.

Interdisciplinary cooperation is basic for tending to muddled, various issues, advancing advancement, and propelling information. Working across disciplines will turn out to be much more significant as the globe gets more interconnected and the difficulties we face become more complicated.

I . Bringing experts from different areas together

Bringing experts from various areas together can bring about development, joint effort, and the creation of novel thoughts. This interdisciplinary strategy is regularly used to tackle convoluted difficulties and move progress in different fields. While uniting experts from different fields, remember the accompanying contemplations:

1. Decide Shared objectives: Guarantee that all experts taking part have a shared objective or issue that should be tended to. This shared objective will be the establishment for association.

2. Various perspectives: Specialists from different callings offer an abundance of information and perspectives of real value. To benefit from this variety, advance open exchange and the trade of thoughts.

3. Lay out clear correspondence courses to overcome any barrier between specialists who might utilize different jargon and ideas. Urge them to communicate their thoughts in manners that others outside their area can comprehend.

4. ability Regard: Perceive and regard every individual's capability. Stay away from pecking orders dependent just upon the subject of study and embrace the worth of different sorts of skill.

5. Facilitation: Consider recruiting a facilitator or middle person to direct discussions, guarantee fair interest, and keep discussions on target toward a shared objective.

6. Interdisciplinary Groups: Structure interdisciplinary groups of individuals from assorted disciplines to team up on unambiguous tasks or hardships. This permits experts to work intently together and use their aggregate information.

7. Critical thinking and Development: Cross-disciplinary joint effort as often as possible outcomes in imaginative thoughts and novel ways to deal with confounded difficulties. Trial and error and innovativeness ought to be supported.

Sharing assets, like gear, information, or assets, can be a successful way to energize interdisciplinary joint efforts and examination.

9. Instruction and Preparing: Permit experts to share their insight. Studios, classes, and preparing occasions can support information move and cross-disciplinary learning.

Archive the cooperative cycle and results. Gather master remarks to work on the cooperation and track down regions for development.

11. Tolerance and Adaptability: Perceive that bringing experts from different areas together may give deterrents and require tolerance. Be versatile and open to new working styles and timetables.

12. Perceive Accomplishments and Achievements: Perceive achievements and achievements to fabricate a feeling of progress and inspiration among the interdisciplinary group.

Uniting experts from numerous areas can be an extraordinary strategy to deal with convoluted issues, advance development, and make critical advances in exploration, innovation, and critical thinking. Powerful correspondence, collaboration, and an eagerness to cooperate toward a solitary goal are required.

Ii. Government and strategy jobs in advancing life span research

In light of multiple factors, the job of government and strategy in supporting life span research is basic. Expanding the human lifetime has significant social, financial, and medical care repercussions, and government commitment can help with the headway of exploration, moral issues, and general well-being.

This position's essential errands are as per the following:

1. Financing and Exploration Backing:

Government bodies, like the Public Foundations of Wellbeing (NIH) in the US, can give huge subsidies to lifespan research. These awards are utilized to help essential exploration, clinical preliminaries, and multidisciplinary studies focused on better grasping the reasons for maturing and making intercessions to advance solid maturing.

2. Oversight and Guideline: Government organizations assume a basic part in managing the turn of events and testing of life span-related medicines and medications. They ensure that examination is directed following moral standards, that security is focused on, and that threats to human subjects are limited.

3. Strategy creation: States can make strategies to help private-area interest in life span research and the formation of related items and administrations. Tax reductions give, and abbreviated administrative strategies for novel medicines are instances of such projects.

4. General Wellbeing programs: Through general wellbeing programs, legislatures can energize great maturing and life span. Missions to advance sound ways of life, successive clinical check-ups, and admittance to safeguard treatment might fall into this classification.

5. Training and Public Mindfulness:
Legislatures might teach people in general about the need for life span research, its expected advantages, and the significance of driving a sound way of life. This can add to the improvement of a culture that values research around here.

6. Information Assortment and Investigation:
Government offices can accumulate and dissect information on maturing and life span to find patterns, difficulties, and open doors. This data can be utilized to direct research needs and strategy choices.

7. Worldwide Joint effort: Participation among state-run administrations and worldwide associations can assist with exploring longer. The sharing of assets, information, and best practices can bring about more effective and fruitful examination results.

8. Moral and Social Contemplations: - States can uphold banters about the moral and social ramifications of life span research, for example, guaranteeing equivalent admittance to medicines and tending to possible errors in medical services access for different populaces.

9. Variation of the Medical Services Framework: State-run administrations might have to change medical services frameworks to meet the necessities of a more established populace as life span research prompts new intercessions and treatments. Changes in medical services conveyance, repayment structures, and long-haul care help might be incorporated.

10. Against Maturing Item Guideline: - Legislatures have some control over and direct the showcasing and offer of against maturing merchandise to shield buyers from deceitful or perilous medicines and to guarantee that any cases made are upheld by logical proof.

Government cooperation in life span research is basic for progressing logical headway, moral contemplations, and the prosperity of maturing populaces. Legislatures might assume a basic part in encouraging comprehension we might interpret as maturing and improving the personal satisfaction for people as they age through subsidizing research, taking on guidelines, and advancing general well-being drives.

Chapter 5

Difficulties and Moral Reflections Concerning Life Expectancy

The longing to draw out human existence term or life expectancy offers challenges and moral situations that ought to be painstakingly thought of. While there might be sure benefits to drawing out human life, there are additionally huge moral and reasonable issues. Here are a few significant worries and moral inquiries regarding life expectancy:

1. Social Dissimilarity: - Challenge: Expanding the typical life expectancy of individuals could exacerbate social and monetary variations because rich individuals would have the option to get life-expansion advances and medicines.

- **Moral Understanding:** To close the hole between the people who can bear the cost of life-saving treatments and the individuals who can't, giving fair admittance to them is fundamental.

2. The cost of clinical consideration could increase later on, particularly for additional laid-out populaces that have higher paces of tenacious contaminations.

- **Moral Reflection**: To adjust the upsides of deferred presence with the monetary weight it will have on medical services frameworks and society, cautious preparation and achievable managerial changes will be required.

3. **Overpopulation**: - Challenge: A significant expansion in the number of individuals in the world could prompt overpopulation, which would place more expectations on regular assets, organic frameworks, and the climate.

- **Moral Understanding:** Techniques for viable populace improvement ought to be looked at throughout related to endeavors to expand human life.

4. Individual delight: - Problem: Expanding the future without focusing on private fulfillment can bring about kept misery or a more unfortunate style of life as one progresses in years.
- **Moral Knowledge**: It is pivotal to ensure that drawn-out care treatments underscore future development in flourishing and prosperity.

5. Resource Assignment: A Troublesome Moral Issue The assignment of resources, like subsidizing for clinical consideration and investigation hypothesis, turns into a complicated moral quandary when life expectancy outweighs other genuine worries about prosperity.
- **Moral Setting**: Fundamental resource part organizing includes adjusting the excursion of a life expectancy with other clinical benefits and cultural worries.

Challenge: Expanding the typical life expectancy of individuals could make accidental impacts, for example, expanding existential dangers like atomic conflict or ecological disaster.

- **Moral Thought**: Moral contemplations ought to take the ramifications of life span for manageability and global security.

7. Individual Freedom: A Test: Assuming that somebody is constrained or restricted as it were, postponing somebody's life might abuse that individual's on the right track to somewhere safe and secure.

- Moral Thought: While choosing which mediations to make to draw out life, it is essential to consider individuals' independence and assent.

8. Mental and Social Impacts: - Challenge: Extending life might introduce mental and social difficulties, like adapting to the death of loved ones or acclimating to social changes.

- Moral Reflection: It is fundamental to prepare society and individuals for the mental and social impacts of longer life expectancies.

9. **Moral Update**: - Issue: Utilizing hereditary or specialized headways to drag out life raises moral worries about being a human and the potential for unseen side effects.
- Moral Idea: Guidelines and management are important to guarantee that life-increasing headways are utilized ethically.

10. **Long haul Impact on Society:** - Challenge: It is hard to foresee the drawn-out impacts of a lot higher futures on normal practices, social idiosyncrasies, and social principles.
- Moral Idea: While making arrangements for longer futures, moral contemplations ought to be considered.

Society must lead fair and taught conversations about these difficulties with a large number of accomplices, lay out moral standards and decide to focus on legislative guidance for people while

likewise uplifting long-lasting learning and
development.

A. Issues with Morals in Life
span Exploration

Research on expanding human existence and
improving personal satisfaction in advanced age
offers different moral conversation starters that
should be appropriately thought out. A portion
of the significant moral problems in life span
research are as per the following:

1. Asset designation: A lot of cash and
individuals are required for life span research.
Burning through cash and assets on life span
research as opposed to squeezing wellbeing and

cultural issues like guaranteeing admittance to essential medical care, disposing of neediness, or battling environmental change makes a moral problem.

2. Value and Access: In the event that life span treatments or medicines become accessible, worries about who gains admittance to these advancements might emerge. Because of the likelihood that inconsistent access could intensify as of now existing social and financial disparities, guaranteeing fair admittance to life span upgrading innovation and therapies is a critical moral concern.

3. Informed Assent: In clinical preliminaries and studies including trial lifespan treatments, getting educated assent can be troublesome, especially while working with senior residents who might have mental weaknesses or restricted skill to settle on conclusions about their wellbeing.

4. unexpected Results: Expanding the typical life expectancy might have unexpected impacts that put more weight on the medical care framework, retirement plans, and regular assets. Scientists should gauge the desire to protract life span against possible unfavorable consequences for society, which could prompt moral situations.

5. Personal satisfaction: As well as zeroing in on life augmentation, life span examination ought to likewise mean to improve personal satisfaction in advanced age. The two objectives can be hard to adjust on the grounds that a few estimates that protect life may not necessarily in every case work on general prosperity.

6. Hereditary Intercessions: The utilization of hereditary intercessions to expand life raises moral worries about changing the human DNA and the chance of accidental impacts, like expanded financial disparity or unexpected medical conditions.

7. Information security and protection: Life span research every now and again involves the get-together and assessment of individual wellbeing data. Concerning the protection of people's delicate data and forestalling its abuse or openness to security breaks, moral scrapes can create.

8. Mental and Cultural Impacts: Carrying on with a more drawn out life can have a negative mental and social effect, for example, making it harder to really focus on others and modifying relational peculiarities. Taking on these issues and setting up reasonable emotionally supportive networks are moral issues.

9. End-of-Life Care: Life span exploration might affect choices about finish-of-life care, for example, when and how to utilize life-augmentation medications instead of palliative consideration. It may very well be troublesome morally to figure out some kind of harmony between the craving for lifespan and the goals of a good passing.

10. Guideline and control: Concluding how much guideline and control is vital for life span exploration and treatments is a continuous moral problem. Finding some kind of harmony between empowering advancement and protecting individuals' security and prosperity is fundamental.

To guarantee that headways in life span benefit society overall while maintaining major moral standards and values, it is essential to painstakingly consider these moral difficulties in life span research. Cooperation between partners is likewise important, as is continuous conversation among scientists, policymakers, ethicists, and the overall population.

I. Judgment of life expansion and personal satisfaction

The confounded test of offsetting life augmentation with personal satisfaction contains moral, clinical, social, and individual variables. As human life expectancies keep on expanding because of clinical and logical advances, individuals and society should consider how to boost both the number and nature of years we live. Here are some significant components to consider while dealing with this equilibrium:

1. Healthspan versus Life expectancy: It means a lot to focus on expanding the time spent living strongly and effectively as opposed to simply extending life overall (life expectancy). The point ought to be to increment both the quantity of years and the quantity of long stretches of life.

2. Clinical Advances: Clinical and biotechnological headways can extend human life expectancies, yet they ought to ideally zero in on forestalling age-related messes and upgrading overall personal satisfaction.

3. Individual Inclinations: Everybody's meaning of personal satisfaction is remarkable and emotional. Others might put a higher need on personal satisfaction than a life span, while some might underscore life span at any expense. Concerning issues regarding individual inclinations and independence is significant.

4. Moral Contemplations: While choosing how to distribute the restricted medical care assets accessible for life expansion, moral difficulties arise. Value and equity should be considered while concluding which individuals get life-augmentation medicines and at what cost.

5. Social and Monetary Ramifications: Expanding the future can have serious social and financial repercussions, for example, an ascent in the requirement for clinical consideration, changes to retirement arrangements, and modifications to benefits frameworks. Conversations of public arrangement should consider these factors.

6. Preventive Medical services: Pushing preventive medical care rehearses like a nutritious eating routine, ordinary activity, and mental prosperity can build life span and personal satisfaction. Age-related issues can be decreased by these activities.

7. Empathy with life care: It's essential to ensure admittance to this sort of care and to regard individuals' finish-of-life inclinations. Zeroing in on an agreeable and noble passing can be similarly basically as urgent as expanding life.

8. Social Associations: Regardless of how long an individual lives, forlornness and social disengagement can adversely affect their satisfaction. The prosperity of more established individuals can be improved by drives to advance social commitment and local area inclusion.

9. Mental Prosperity: Further developing psychological well-being issues like nervousness and sadness is fundamental for safeguarding a great life as individuals age. Alongside actual well-being, advancing psychological well-being ought to be a top objective.

10. Comprehensive Methodologies: Adopt into account comprehensive strategies for well-being and prosperity, for example, mind-body practices like care, yoga, and contemplation, which can upgrade both physical and mental prosperity.

A multidisciplinary approach and open correspondence between individuals, medical care experts, legislators, and ethicists are important to effectively offset life expansion with personal satisfaction. Assisting people with living longer, better lives while regarding their convictions and choices concerning the sort of life they wish to seek in their later years ought to be a definitive goal.

Ii. Approaching Novel life span treatments

It's a muddled and creating issue to gain admittance to new life span cures. The objective of life span medicines is to protect human existence and improve general well-being and prosperity in advanced age. Operations, dietary changes, and biotechnological progressions are a couple of instances of these medicines. Here are some significant things to contemplate with openness to novel lifespan medicines:

1. Innovative work: Numerous enemies of maturing treatments are as of now in the testing or starter transformative phases. Just the people who are signed up for clinical preliminaries or who have specific clinical issues that qualify them for exploratory treatment might gain admittance to these drugs.

2. Administrative Endorsement: Before being made broadly accessible, any lifespan treatment should typically pass severe testing and get an administrative endorsement from associations like the European Meds Office (EMA) or the U.S. Food and Medication Organization (FDA). This strategy could happen for quite a long time.

3. Treatment Accessibility: Following administrative leeway, a lifespan treatment's openness might contrast by region and medical services framework. Access might be affected by things like expenses, insurance inclusion, and clinical contracts.

4. Price: The cost of new lifespan medicines can be a significant access hindrance. Especially for trial or elective activities, a few treatments could be costly, and healthcare coverage inclusion may be scant or nonexistent.

Admittance to state-of-the-art lifespan medicines can exacerbate medical care. accessibility to these therapies might be simpler for specific individuals than for other people, contingent upon their monetary circumstances or accessibility to the state-of-the-art clinical offices.

6. Moral Contemplations: There are moral predicaments around who ought to approach life span prescriptions and under what conditions. A troublesome undertaking is guaranteeing fair access while considering the benefits and weaknesses that can exist.

7. Way of life and Preventive Measures: It's a memorable fundamental that numerous life expectancy increments can be achieved through way-of-life changes and preventive measures, for example, maintaining a reasonable eating regimen, routine work-out, and swearing off dangerous propensities like smoking and unnecessary drinking. Most individuals can frequently acquire these intercessions.

8. Life span as an area: The life span region is rapidly creating, and discoveries are being made constantly. Access might increment on the off chance that more medicines become open as exploration propels.

9. Counseling Clinical Specialists: Individuals who are keen on state-of-the-art life span cures ought to talk with clinical specialists who can exhort them on the latest examination, clinical preliminaries, and benefits and inconveniences.

Factors including the phase of examination, administrative endorsement, cost, medical care strategy, and moral issues all affect how available new lifespan therapies are. Even though there is a rising interest in expanding human existence and upgrading well-being in advanced age, admittance to these treatments might be limited and may vary depending upon one's area and individual conditions. While pondering life span mediations, it's pivotal to stay aware of leap forwards in the field and look for master direction.

B. The Monetary and Social Impacts of Life span Treatment

The social and monetary repercussions of life span treatments, which mean to increment human life span and improve personal satisfaction in advanced age, are multifaceted and different. While there are numerous potential benefits, for example, more seasoned individuals who are better and more useful, there are likewise challenges and potential adverse consequences that should be considered. Here are a few significant contemplations:

Good cultural and monetary repercussions

1. More prominent Efficiency of the Labor force: Individuals' functioning lives might be drawn out assuming that life span medicines assist them with remaining sound and dynamic for longer. This might reduce work deficiencies, ease monetary strain welcomed on by retirement, and advance financial extension.

2. Lower Clinical Expenses: By stopping or deferring the beginning old enough related ailments and incapacities, life span medicines

might diminish the burden on medical services frameworks. Better individuals need less long-haul care and clinical mediation, which could bring about less expensive medical services costs.

3. Expanded Open doors for Mastering and Expertise Obtaining: Individuals who live longer might have additional time and impetus to seek extra schooling and preparation, bringing about a more talented and versatile labor force.

4. Expanded Saving and Effective Financial Planning: Individuals might be more propelled to save and contribute on the off chance that they expect to carry on with a more extended life, which could bring about more capital collection and monetary dependability.

5. Advancement and Exploration: The quest for lifespan cures might prod academic and clinical requests, potentially bringing about advancements in biotechnology and medical services that are beneficial to society at large.

Adverse results and Hindrances

1. Monetary Supportability: As additional people depend on these projects for a more extended period, a more drawn-out future populace might put weight on the social government assistance and benefits frameworks. The monetary practicality of such projects should be tended to by policymakers.

2. Pay Imbalance: If simply a part of the populace can bear the cost of life-span medicines, pay, and well-being disparities might deteriorate because of the inconsistent dissemination of admittance to these medicines and the advantages they give.

3. Overpopulation: On the off chance that a significantly longer life expectancy isn't joined by lower rates of birth, it could bring about overpopulation, which would overwhelm the climate's assets.

Longer life expectancies might require adjustments to family game plans, cultural norms, and retirement anticipations. The thoughts of legacy and generational progression could likewise be impacted.

5. Moral Issues: The accessibility and utilization of life-span medicines make moral issues, for example, who ought to approach, how medicines ought to be administered, and what are the ramifications for end-of-life decisions.

6. Monetary Interruption: Stretched life ranges might change conventional retirement and business design creating an awkward nature in the work market and intergenerational clashes.

7. Long haul Medical services Expenses: While lifespan therapies might save some medical services costs in the close to term, they might bring about higher long haul medical services costs as individuals might require more escalated and concentrated care as they age.

The imminent impacts on society and the economy of life-span medicines may be both advantageous and terrible. Policymakers, medical services experts, and society as the need might arise to have smart discussions ponder the moral ramifications, and plan completely for the turn of events, dissemination, and impact of such therapies to expand the advantages and reduce the hindrances. A difficult and progressing undertaking will be finding some kind of harmony between the craving for longer and better lives and monetary correspondence and supportability.

I . Longer futures and their consequences for medical care and retirement frameworks

Worldwide retirement and medical care frameworks are fundamentally affected by longer life expectancies. Indeed, even while better medical services and everyday environments by and large lead to longer life expectancies, a few issues should be settled.

1. Rising Retirement Expenses: - Individuals spend more years in retirement because of living longer. This overburdens retirement frameworks, eminently on government managed retirement and conventional characterized benefit annuity plans. These frameworks could require funding or changes to help retired people for a more drawn out time span.

Worries about maintainability: A critical test is the lifespan of retirement frameworks. Less supporters might be accessible to help every retired person if the extent of retired people to individuals of working age rises. This might bring about supporting holes and the necessity for changes to ensure the drawn out feasibility of these frameworks.

3. Medical services costs: Higher medical care costs are in many cases a symptom of longer life expectancies since more established individuals are bound to encounter age-related medical conditions. This rising interest for medical care administrations can possibly put a weight on public medical services frameworks and drive up costs for the two residents and legislatures.

4. Age-Related Illnesses: Longer life expectancies increment the gamble of creating age-related sicknesses and persistent afflictions like Alzheimer's infection, diabetes, and cardiovascular illnesses. It takes specific treatment and backing to address specific medical problems, which could raise medical care costs.

5. Labor force Suggestions: - Expanding life expectancies could require adjusting retirement ages and labor force support. The retirement age has previously been expanded in certain countries to help their retirement plans. Longer working vocations for more established individuals could assist with diminishing the monetary cost that accompanies living longer.

6. Long haul Care Necessities: Expanded interest for long haul care administrations, like nursing homes and home medical services, is regularly a consequence of longer life expectancies. These administrations can be expensive, which expands the weight on medical services frameworks and families to really focus on the older.

The need to get ready for longer retirements might require more prominent speculations and reserve funds in retirement accounts.
7. Monetary Arranging Difficulties. To ensure that individuals can support themselves

adequately in advanced age, monetary schooling and proficiency become urgent.

8. Intergenerational Value: Because of longer life expectancies, there might be stresses over intergenerational value, as more youthful ages might be compelled to bear an uncalled for portion of the expense of supporting the old through duties and commitments to retirement plans.

States, partnerships, and people should step up and resolve these issues. Transforming the retirement and medical services frameworks, encouraging sound maturing and safeguarding medical care, advancing expanded labor force commitment, and helping with retirement monetary arranging are a couple of instances of what this can involve. The impacts of longer life expectancies on these frameworks can likewise be made do with the guide of savvy fixes like public-private associations and innovation driven medical services.

Ii. Dispensing with contrasts in life span results

A blend of legislative, medical services, financial, and social mediations is expected to address the distinctions in life span results since it is a mind-boggling and multi-layered subject. These errors habitually reflect hidden social determinants of well-being, including financial status, level of instruction, admittance to mind, and local area conditions. Coming up next are a few strategies and thoughts to address these differences:

Admittance to and nature of medical services - Widespread Medical care: Guarantee that everybody approaches quality, reasonable medical services, regardless of their financial circumstance.

1 - Medical care Value: Set up arrangements and practices that elevate fair admittance to clinical benefits, including screenings, protection care, and medicines.

2. Medical care for Anticipation: Advanced well-being schooling and proficiency in minimized populaces to bring issues to light of sound ways of life and ailment avoidance.

Support people with group-based drives that give an accentuation on dietary propensities, actual work, and sound way of life choices.

3. Tending to social determinants of well-being, including measures like living compensation, open lodging, and occupation preparation, can assist with diminishing financial uniqueness and further develop business possibilities.
- Schooling: Put resources into top-notch training, particularly in underestimated regions, to upgrade financial versatility and long-haul well-being results.
Increment admittance to healthy, sensibly valued food choices, especially in food deserts, and backing drives that teach individuals about nourishment.

Changes to the Medical Care Framework
Preparing medical care experts in social ability and aversion to the requirements of changed networks.
- Information Social occasion and Investigation: Assemble and look at disparities

in well-being information to pinpoint and address specific requirements.

5. Local area Strengthening: Include nearby networks in navigation and medical care wanting to ensure that administrations match their specific prerequisites.
- Steady Organizations: Energize socially encouraging groups of people that can offer consistent encouragement and commonsense assistance to individuals managing well-being incongruities.

5. Actual Wellbeing and Health:
- Emotional well-being Administrations: Extend admittance to psychological well-being care, particularly in minimized regions, to address the association between stress and poor psychological wellness and abbreviated future. Send off the enemy of shame projects to urge individuals to look for care and to reduce the disgrace related to psychological wellness conditions.

7. Socially Skilled Treatment: - Different Medical services Labor force: Grow variety among medical care experts to convey socially capable therapy and reduce inclination.
- Language Access: Guarantee that deterrents to getting to medical care administrations because of language are taken out.

8. Strategy and Backing: - Legislation: Advance regulations and strategies that arrange wellbeing imbalances and advance value in medical care.
- Exploration and Assessment: Empower concentrates on examining the basic factors that add to differences and evaluate the viability of medicines.

9. Collaboration and Unions: Empower participation between medical services suppliers, local area associations, legislative associations, and beneficent associations to create comprehensive arrangements.

10. Media missions to bring issues to light of issues: To acquire support for projects tending to well-being aberrations, and increment public information on these issues and their belongings.

A continuous responsibility from legislatures, medical services organizations, networks, and people is expected to address disparities in life expectancy results. Building an all the more impartial society where everybody gets the opportunity to carry on with a long and solid life, involves both quick fixes and central changes.

C . Guideline and wellbeing stresses over the drawn out results

Since they incorporate tending to the potential risks and moral inquiries raised by treatments intended to extend human lifetime, administrative and wellbeing issues connected with life span results are complicated and multi-layered. Administrative and security issues are special to each kind of life span examination and intercession, which could go from dietary changes to bleeding edge biotechnological improvements. Following are a few significant issues:

1. Moral and Social Ramifications: Life span research raises moral worries about the appropriation of assets, admittance to life-augmentation innovation, and the potential for exacerbated imbalance. decisions about who

gets these intercessions and how they are scattered are vital.

2. Clinical Wellbeing: To ensure its security, any operation expected to increment human life span should go through broad clinical testing. To assess the possible risks and advantages as well as any unforeseen incidental effects, extended preliminaries are often essential.

3. Guideline and Endorsement: Administrative associations like the U.S. Food and Medication Organization (FDA) are crucial for the assessment and endorsement of life span treatments. The inclination for development should be offset with guaranteeing wellbeing and viability, which is a ceaseless issue.

4. Logical Legitimacy: The proof supporting various treatments to advance lifespan is as yet created. Given the intricacy and multi-faceted nature of the maturing system, characterizing what considers solid logical proof for these intercessions can be troublesome.

5. Information security and protection:
Assembling and dissecting private wellbeing
data is a typical move toward life span research.
To safeguard individuals' privileges and stop
abuse, guaranteeing the protection and security
of this data is fundamental.

6. Long haul influences: Since the point is to
increment lifetime, assessing the drawn out
effects of interventions is pivotal. To really
comprehend the effect on wellbeing and life
span, noticing individuals over an extensive
period might be vital.

7. Monetary Issues: The expense of examination,
improvement, and treatment access for life span
treatments can be high. To forestall laying out
medical services disparities, the estimating and
availability of these mediations should be
considered.

8. Psychosocial Effect: Expanding the typical
life expectancy of individuals might have mental

and social repercussions, for example, the chance of a maturing populace overburdening medical care frameworks, retirement plans, and other cultural designs.

9. Administrative Holes: To keep up with appropriate observing, it could be important to fill administrative holes as new life span treatments are created.

10. undesirable Impacts: Expanding life expectancy might have undesirable impacts like populace development, a higher ecological strain, or unexpected cultural changes.

11. Misrepresentation and Bogus Data: Attempting to carry on with a long life might draw in scalawags and support the spread of bogus data. To defend the general population against tricky promoting and hazardous items, administrative bodies should practice cautiousness.

12. Global Participation: Since life span research is a worldwide undertaking, there is a requirement for global participation and the harmonization of administrative prerequisites to ensure consistency and security across borders.

For the proper exploration and execution of treatments expected to broaden the human lifetime, it is vital to address these administrative and wellbeing concerns. As life span research is created, it will turn out to be harder to figure out some kind of harmony between empowering advancement, shielding individuals, and considering moral and cultural issues.

I. Guaranteeing the life span and security of meds against maturing

It is urgent to guarantee a singular's security and reasonability since hostile to development mediations much of the time address the normal patterns of development and essentially affect a singular's prosperity and flourishing. A couple of critical components and activities that can assist with ensuring the security and suitability of such interventions are recorded beneath:

1. Imaginative work: Carry out severe preclinical groundwork: Any enemy of developing a drug ought to go through exhaustive preclinical testing in research center circumstances before being utilized on people. Testing for cells, creatures, or other applicable models is important to figure out its parts and any risks.

   - Inspect the basics of science: Understanding the natural maturing cycle of the body is fundamental. While planning intercessions, experts ought to focus on recognizing the exact targets and pathways connected with development.

2. Clinical assessments: Stage 1 assessments: To measure the intervention's security, peace, and adverse consequences, begin with restricted scope human fundamental examinations.

To start assessing practicality and go on with security assessments, Stage 2 fundamental gatherings ought to be extended to incorporate bigger gatherings.

- Stage 3 starter studies: Lead huge, randomized, twofold visually impaired evaluations of outwardly impeded individuals to check their well-being and practicality across a scope of populaces.

Long haul follow-up Whenever they have passed the assessment, watch out for any primer individuals to search for any potential security blemishes or guarantee results.

3. Moral reflections: Before partaking in clinical assessments, ensure individuals are educated about the dangers and benefits regarding the intercession and give their educated assent.

   - Try not to play the two sides: Moral standards ought to guarantee that impeded social events are not exploited and that all gatherings go to intervention.

4. Managerial Oversight: In the US, managerial associations like the FDA (Food and Medicine Association) expect a key job in surveying and embracing hostility to developing prescriptions. To analyze the security and reasonability of the medications, they assess information from clinical fundamental examinations.

5. Peer Review: Before being distributed in trustworthy legitimate diaries, the examination ought to go through a cautious companion review to ensure the nature and validity of the outcomes.

6. Transparency: Experts and associations ought to be transparent about their techniques, discoveries, and possibly unsound conditions to hold authenticity and confirmation.

7. Progress Checking: The facts confirm that the enemy of maturing drugs ought to be assessed for their drawn-out viability and reasonableness, and any regrettable secondary effects ought to be expected and expeditiously managed, even after getting approval.

8. Customized Medication: Know that only one out of every odd medication will altogether impact each individual. Upgraded strategies might be important to further develop benefits and diminish gambles considering acquired characteristics, way of life, and different variables.

9. Instruction and Public Care: - Illuminate the overall population about the advantages and downsides of threatening to develop

interventions to help with pursuing very educated choices.

10. Look at assumptions by focusing on the way that the counter-development treatment can't deliver moments or heavenly advantages and that development is a mind-boggling cycle with a large number.

By and large, guaranteeing the security and viability of hostile to maturing prescriptions requires a full and convoluted framework that incorporates cautious investigation, moral worries, regulatory oversight, and steady insight. This cycle is fundamental to safeguard individuals and to examine research that is unsafe to develop.

Ii. How administrative offices assume a part in management

Administrative associations can assist with watching out for worries connected with life span, particularly in businesses where they have a major effect. In this sense, the expression "life span" alludes to the difficulties and amazing open doors that accompany an expansion in the normal human life expectancy. Here are a few different ways that administrative offices could supervise life span:

1. Biomedical Exploration and Drugs: Administrative associations like the European Meds Organization (EMA) and the U.S. Food and Medication Organization (FDA) oversee the examination and endorsement of meds and treatments that are planned to extend solid lives or treat age-related messes. Before being advertised to the overall population, they assess the well-being and viability of such mediations.

2. Clinical Gadgets: Administrative bodies likewise watch out for the creation and utilization of clinical gadgets that are connected with life span, like embedded gadgets or geriatric consideration analytic gear. They ensure these devices stick to execution and security prerequisites.

3. Nursing Homes and Senior Consideration: In the space of senior consideration, administrative associations watch out for nursing homes and help residing offices to ensure they offer legitimate consideration and stick to lawful prerequisites for the prosperity of more established occupants.

4. Medical care Access: Administrative associations might address worries about medical services access and moderation, which might affect the norm of care for older individuals. They could make guidelines to work with more established individuals' admittance to medical care administrations.

5. Protection and Monetary Administrations: Administrative bodies in the monetary business might be accountable for protection items like annuities or long haul care protection that are planned to address lifespan issues. They ensure that these monetary items are simple and give policyholders their normal benefits.

6. Research morals: Moral issues in lifespan research are significant. Specifically, in fields like human life expectancy expansion or hereditary treatments, administrative specialists might be engaged with directing the ethical lead of examination including people.

7. Information insurance and protection: Since gathering and breaking down delicate well-being information is a typical piece of life-span research, administrative associations might play a part in maintaining information security and security regulations to safeguard the individual information of exploration members.

8. Public getting it and Schooling:
Administrative bodies might work with different gatherings to provide additional government-funded training and understanding on issues connecting with life span, maturing, and medical services. This can include teaching individuals about assets and great maturing ways of behaving.

9. Personal satisfaction Guidelines: In certain circumstances, administrative associations might lay out prerequisites for the consideration and personal satisfaction of old individuals, considering factors like lodging, transportation, and social help administrations.

10. Research Subsidizing and Awards:
Administrative associations oftentimes give research subsidizing and awards to help learn about life expectancy. The command over how these assets are dispensed and utilized might be practiced by administrative specialists.

It's important that relying upon the country, the district, and the administrative office's specific area of focus, the job of administrative associations in controlling lifespan could vary. Moreover, the investigation of life span is growing rapidly, and administrative methodologies might change because of new logical discoveries as well as rising moral and cultural issues. Generally speaking, administrative organizations can be critical in guaranteeing that headway in the subject of life span is protected, moral, and favorable to the two individuals and society overall.

Chapter 6

Contextual analyses and Examples of overcoming adversity

Life span contextual investigations and examples of overcoming adversity much of the time include people or gatherings who have carried on with exceptional lives, which are for the most part connected to a blend of way of life elements, hereditary qualities, and medical services. The following are a couple of renowned models:

1. Blue Zones: Blue Zones are regions all over the planet where individuals reside significantly longer, and better. Okinawa (Japan), Sardinia (Italy), the Nicoya Landmass (Costa Rica), Ikaria (Greece), and Loma Linda (California, USA) are among these areas. Scientists have explored these spots to more readily figure out the shared characteristics among their populaces.

Plant-based, major areas of strength for diet connections, ordinary active work, and low feelings of anxiety are habitually distinguished as adding to life span in these societies.

2. Jeanne Calment: Jeanne Calment holds the Guinness World Record for the most established affirmed human life span, having lived to the age of 122 years and 164 days. She credited her life span to an eating routine wealthy in olive oil, port wine, and chocolate, as well as being dynamic and keeping a cheerful outlook.

3. Mbah Gotho: An Indonesian man named Mbah Gotho professed to be the world's most established individual, with proof demonstrating he was 146 years of age when he passed on in 2017. Although his age has been tested, his account has caused him to notice the need for right-birth endorsements and the opportunities for uncommon life.

4. Emma Morano: Emma Morano was an Italian lady who lived to be 117 years of age, making

her perhaps the most established individual in recorded history. She credited her long life to an ordinary eating routine of crude eggs and treats, as well as hereditary qualities and a tranquil way of life.

5. Centenarian Investigations: A few investigations have focused on centenarians (individuals who live to the age of 100 or more) to find the mysteries of their life span. These examinations often find that hereditary qualities play a significant impact, however solid way of life decisions like a decent eating regimen, exercise, and social inclusion likewise add to their long lives.

6. Caloric Limitation: Creature studies have shown that caloric limitation, or restricting calorie admission without unhealthiness, can increment life expectancy. While the review is as yet in progress, it has provoked revenue in researching the potential advantages of calorie limitation in people.

7. Public Life span Drives: Nations, for example, Japan and Singapore have laid out public drives to advance sound maturing and increment the number of centenarians. These tasks now and again incorporate medical services progress, social exercises, and guidelines zeroed in on supporting more established populaces.

8. Hereditary Disclosures: Progresses in hereditary qualities have found explicit hereditary variations associated with improved life span. The APOE quality, for instance, has been connected with life span, for certain changes happening all the more normally in centenarians.

These contextual investigations and examples of overcoming adversity exhibit the changed idea of life span, with hereditary qualities, way of life, and ecological factors all having an impact. While there is no one size-fits-all remedy for carrying on with a long life, these models give an understanding of the propensities and conditions that can add to a more extended, better life expectancy.

People Who Have Achieved Remarkable Life span

Uncommon life span is much of the time portrayed as living to the age of 100 or more established. It is an astonishing achievement to live such a long and solid life. The following are a couple of individuals who have carried on with extraordinarily lengthy lives and become popular for their age:

1. Jeanne Calment (1875-1997): Jeanne Calment of France is one of the most notable instances of a wonderful life span. She lived to be 122 years and 164 days old, making her the most established confirmed person in written history.

2. Sarah Knauss (1880-1999): Sarah Knauss was an American lady who lived to the age of 119 years and 97 days. She was the world's most established living individual when she kicked the bucket.

3. Jiroemon Kimura (1897-2013): Jiroemon Kimura, a Japanese man, is quite possibly the longest-living man in written history. long term and 54 days on the planet.

4. Susannah Mushatt Jones (1899-2016): Susannah Mushatt Jones, an American lady,

turned into the world's most seasoned living individual in 2015, living to the age of 116 years and 311 days.

5. Emma Morano (1899-2017): Emma Morano, an Italian lady, was one of the last individuals brought into the world in the nineteenth century.117 years and 137 days she lived.

6. Nabi Tajima (1900-2018): Nabi Tajima, a Japanese lady, turned into the world's most established living individual in 2018 at 117 years old and 260 days.

7. Kane Tanaka (conceived 1903): Kane Tanaka, likewise from Japan, is the world's most established living individual as of September 2021. She was brought into the world in 1903 and has been known for her phenomenal life span.

Kindly remember that carrying on with such a long life regularly requires a blend of hereditary qualities, way-of-life decisions, and admittance to medical services.

I.Perspectives from centenarians and supercentenarians

Centenarians and supercentenarians (the individuals who live to arrive at 100 years of age) have long drawn in specialists because of their surprising life expectancy. While there is no one-size-fits-all procedure for carrying on with a long life, bits of knowledge from these people can give critical examples to those hoping to carry on with a more extended, better life. Here are a few significant bits of knowledge from centenarians and supercentenarians:

1. Hereditary qualities Have an Effect: Hereditary qualities can fundamentally affect life span. Certain individuals might acquire hereditary attributes that make them more impervious to specific illnesses or further develop life span. Scientists have recognized specific qualities associated with life span, for example, the FOXO3 quality, which has been connected to a more drawn-out lifetime.

2. Way-of-life Decisions Matter: While hereditary qualities have an influence, way-of-life decisions significantly affect life expectancy. A huge number stress the meaning of driving a sound way of life, which incorporates eating a reasonable eating routine, outstanding, truly dynamic, not smoking, and restricting liquor consumption.

3. Social connections: Solid social connections and a feeling of the local area are habitually

viewed as fundamental determinants of life span. Keeping up close bonds with loved ones can offer profound help and lower pressure, the two of which can add to carrying on with a more drawn-out life.

4. Uplifting perspective: A positive perspective on life is connected with upgraded well-being and life expectancy. Indeed, despite difficulty, a huge number and supercentenarians keep a constant and confident viewpoint.

5. Sustenance is Significant: Sustenance is a significant piece of carrying on with a long and solid life. A huge number consume fewer calories that underline new food sources, vegetables, and natural products while decreasing handled food sources, sugar, and soaked fats. The Mediterranean eating routine, which incorporates a lot of olive oil, fish, and new produce, is much of the time suggested as a smart dieting design.

6. Active work: Customary actual work is critical for general well-being and life expectancy. A large number take part in regular actual side interests like strolling, cultivating, or kendo, which keep them dynamic and portable.

7. Stress The board: Since stress can hurt one's well-being, great pressure on the board is fundamental. Centenarians as often as possible use pressure-decreasing methods like contemplation, yoga, and care.

8. Scholarly Commitment: Mental well-being should keep up with mental action. A large number keep on participating in intellectually animating side interests like perusing, riddles, or gaining new abilities.

9. flexibility: Adaptability and adaptability despite life's difficulties are vital attributes for life span. Centenarians oftentimes show steadiness and the capacity to adapt to difficulty.

10. Customary Well Being Tests: A huge number underscore the requirement for ordinary clinical tests and preventive medical care. Early identification and treatment of well-being problems can work on by and large personal satisfaction and increment life span.

It's urgent to note that singular variables and conditions differ, and not all centenarians experience the same way. Life span is the result of a mind-boggling connection between hereditary qualities, climate, way of life, and karma. While these experiences can be helpful, there are no certifications concerning carrying on with a long and sound life. In any case, driving a solid way of life and keeping magnificent social connections can essentially expand one's possibilities of living in a mature age.

Ii. Their life span mysteries

The life expectancy of centenarians (the people who live to be 100 or more seasoned) and supercentenarians (the individuals who live to be 110 or more seasoned) captivates the two specialists and the overall population. While there is no single "secret" to their life span, a few factors are generally connected with their extensive life expectancies. It is pivotal to take note that hereditary qualities have an immense impact in deciding how long somebody can live, yet way-of-life decisions likewise assume a part. Here are a few critical components that might add to the lifespan of centenarians and supercentenarians:

1. Genetics: Hereditary qualities assume a fundamental part in impacting life span. Certain individuals are hereditarily inclined toward carrying on with longer lives because of factors, for example, diminished vulnerability to progress in years-related illnesses or more slow maturing processes.

2. Solid Eating routine: A large number and supercentenarians eat an eating regimen high in natural products, vegetables, solid grains, and lean proteins. They often eat an even eating regimen that is low in handled food sources and high in sugar.

3. Actual work: Ordinary active work is connected to life span. To remain dynamic, a huge number take part in low-influence exercises like strolling, planting, or yoga.

4. Psychological wellness: It is basic to Keep up with amazing psychological wellness. Remaining intellectually connected through

exercises like riddles or perusing, as well as controlling pressure, can all assist you with carrying on with a more extended life.

5. Strong social connections: Having a strong emotionally supportive network and keeping social connections with loved ones will further develop a life span. Everyday reassurance and a feeling of having a place are imperative.

6. No Smoking: Most centenarians and supercentenarians are nonsmokers or stopped smoking when they were young. Smoking is a significant gambling factor for some age-related messes.

7. Moderate Liquor Utilization: A few centenarians report moderate liquor utilization, especially red wine, which might have cardiovascular advantages. Inordinate liquor use, then again, is unsafe for one's well-being.

8. hopeful Disposition: A hopeful mentality toward life and the capacity to adjust to changes

and difficulties can prompt a more drawn-out, more blissful life.

9. Staying away from Unreasonable Pressure: Stress the board practices, for example, reflection or yoga can work on broad well-being.

10. Customary Check-Ups: A large number and supercentenarians esteem normal clinical check-ups and preventive medical services, which can recognize and address medical problems early.

11. Staying away from Weight: Keeping a solid body weight throughout life is fundamental for life expectancy. Heftiness is a significant gamble factor for an assortment of medical problems.

12. Sufficient and Peaceful Rest: Satisfactory and serene rest is basic for general well-being. A huge number report having ordinary resting designs.

13. Restricted Prescription Use: A few centenarians have had little openness to meds all

through their lifetimes, particularly if they have kept away from constant circumstances.

It is basic to grasp that not all centenarians and supercentenarians stick to these standards precisely and that there is no one-size-fits-all recipe for lifespan. Hereditary elements, natural factors, and karma all have an influence. Regardless, taking on a sound way of life that incorporates these standards can expand your possibilities of carrying on with a more drawn-out and better life.

B.Institutions and Drives Advancing Life span

Advancing life span and solid maturing has been fundamentally important for some establishments and projects all over the planet. These associations and tries are devoted to propelling examination, training, and authoritative changes to increment human life expectancy and work on personal satisfaction in advanced age. Here are a few critical establishments and tasks that advance lifespan:

1. Sens Exploration Establishment: This non-benefit association is devoted to the turn of events and advancement of regenerative medication medicines to fight maturing. They work to fix the harm that occurs at the cell and subatomic levels to stretch a sound lifetime.

2. Life span Vision Asset: This funding store puts resources into organizations and tasks that are making advances and treatments to increment human life span, like the enemy of maturing drugs, biotechnology, and computerized well-being arrangements.

3. Calico (California Life business): An auxiliary of Letters in Order Inc. (Google's parent business), Calico is committed to researching the science of maturing and making answers to expand human existence. They work with different scholastic organizations and biotech firms.

4. Buck Establishment for Exploration on Maturing: This independent exploration foundation centers exclusively around maturing and age-related messes. They examine to all the more likely grasp the science of maturing and formulate methodologies to advance sound maturing.

5. Public Establishment on Maturing (NIA): Part of the Public Foundations of Wellbeing (NIH) in the US, the NIA is focused on maturing research. They support and carry out analysis to all the more likely grasp the maturing system and foster answers for expanding one's well-being.

6. European Development Organization on Dynamic and Solid Maturing (EIP-AHA): This European Association program unites partners from numerous enterprises to cultivate advancement in dynamic and solid maturing. It advances exploration, development, and strategy improvement.

7. World Wellbeing Association (WHO) Maturing and Wellbeing System: The WHO advances solid maturing universally using exploration, backing, and strategy creation. They work in age-accommodating environmental factors, staying away from age-related illnesses, and empowering admittance to medical services for more established people.

8. American League for Maturing Exploration (Far off): Far off advances and supports research on maturing and age-related messes. They give awards and assets to researchers chipping away at drives focused on drawing out human life expectancies and expanding personal satisfaction in advanced age.

Human Lifespan, Inc.: Established by genomics pioneer Craig Venter, this organization centers around genomics and information-driven ways to deal with figuring out the science of maturing. They give well-being assessments and genomic sequencing administrations to help individuals control their well-being and life span.

10. Life span Gatherings and Meetings: Different gatherings and discussions, like the Life span Discussion and the Maturing Exploration and Medication Disclosure Meeting, unite trained professionals, scientists, and policymakers to discuss maturing-related subjects and drives.

These foundations and projects are basic in propelling examination, innovation, and strategy pointed toward drawing out life span and working on the personal satisfaction for maturing populaces. They work with researchers, policymakers, and the business area to propel the study of maturing and life span.

I.Notable life span research foundations and gatherings

There are a few critical life span research offices and gatherings all over the planet committed to examining and expanding human life expectancy. The following are a few models:

1. The Buck Organization for Exploration on Maturing: Situated in Novato, California, the Buck Foundation is one of the world's head research offices zeroed in on maturing and age-related messes. They embrace state-of-the-art research on the science of maturing to foster treatments to expand health span and life expectancy.

2. Sens Exploration Establishment: Dr. Aubrey de Dim shaped this philanthropic establishment to explore and elevate regenerative medication answers to address the center's reasons for

maturing. They support research activities and cooperate with different associations to speed the advancement of medicines that can increment the human lifespan.

3. Life span Vision Asset: The Life span Vision Asset is a funding firm that puts resources into organizations and innovations that can enormously drag out human existence. They reserve endeavors and exploration projects in the domain of life span and maturing.

4. The Life Expectancy Organization at the College of Southern California: This exploration office, connected with the USC Leonard Davis School of Gerontology, attempts multidisciplinary research on maturing and life expectancy. They need to figure out the atomic underpinnings of maturing and think up methodologies to advance solid maturing.

5. Harvard T.H. Chan School of General Wellbeing - Community for Life Span Review: Harvard's Middle for Life Span Studies is

devoted to promoting the study of solid maturing. They concentrate on the social, monetary, and well-being parts of life span and maturing.

6. Max Planck Organization for Science of Maturing: Situated in Cologne, Germany, this foundation concentrates on the atomic reasons for maturing. They investigate the hereditary and cell components that add to maturing and search for answers to increment solid life expectancy.

7. Science of Maturing Research Center at the École Polytechnique Fédérale de Lausanne (EPFL): This Swiss exploration lab is committed to grasping the science of maturing and age-related messes. They are focusing on treatments that could expand health span and life expectancy.

8. Buckingham Royal Residence Organization of Life span: This UK-based organization partnered with Buckingham Castle plans to speed up examination into maturing and life span. They

work with chief researchers and organizations to build how we might interpret maturing and foster novel medicines.

The Public Organization on Maturing (NIA): The Public Organizations of Wellbeing (NIH) is an administration body focused on maturing research. They support a large number of concentrates on maturing, well-being, and life span.

10. The Life span Consortium: This cooperative undertaking unites specialists from numerous foundations to team up on grasping the hereditary and sub-atomic underpinnings of maturing. They need to find new treatment focuses to assist people in living longer, better lives.

These organizations and exploration focuses assume basic parts in extending how we might interpret maturing and formulating systems to advance solid maturing and increment human lifetime. If it's not too much trouble, remember that the scene of life span research is continually changing, so there might be other creating focuses and associations also.

Ii. The commitment of eminent future examination centers around life-length research

A couple of conspicuous future explorations concentrated generally throughout the globe have made enormous interests in the field of future and the assessment of evaluating human life trust. Some of them, close by their wonderful obligations, are according to the accompanying:

1. The Buck Relationship for Examination of Maternity (USA): - Driven research at work of cell senescence in developing and advancement-related issues.
- overseen assessment of the impact of calorie limits and clashing fasting in the future.
- Pondered using senolytic medicines to perceive and clear out senescent cells.

2. Salk Beginning stage for Normal Appraisals (USA): Driven escalated assessment on the

revelation of the counter-developing molecule telomerase.
- Explored the ability of telomeres, the guarded covers on the completions of chromosomes, in developing and sickness.
- Investigated the logical effects of medications that increase telomeres.

3. Harvard T.H. Chan School of General Success (USA): - Driven critical assessment on lifestyle parts like food, exercise, and social ties that increase future.
- Specialists assess the heritability of the future through examinations of centenarians and their families.

4. The School of Cambridge Future Science Program (UK) examined the investigation of improvement and the future, recognizing different qualities connected with an extraordinary future.
- analyzed how biological factors — like air quality and money-related situations — impact development.

5. Max Planck Relationship for Investigation of Creating (Germany): Driven research on the investigation of creating, focusing on work of mitochondria, energetic life forms, and metabolic pathways.
- explored the effects of calorie limits and dietary upgrades from here on out.

6. Relationship for Mature Examination, Albert Einstein School of Prescription (USA): - Examined the science behind issues connected with developing, similar to osteoporosis and Alzheimer's disease.
- Investigated the responsibility of inborn and epigenetic variables for improvement.

The US Solid Creating and Future Examination Establishment is arranged at the School of Washington Prescription.
- Managed examination concerning the effects of unsettling influence and safe framework breakdown on improvement.

- Examined immunotherapies' ability to broaden life and further foster prosperity.

8. Barshop Beginning stage for Future and Creating Examinations, UT Prosperity San Antonio (USA): - Examined the genetic and cell patterns of creating with an accentuation on senescence and DNA fix.
- Researched expected results of life-growing steady intercessions.

9. Different areas of insulin medication
- Searched for potential prescriptions for extending the future using electronic thinking and man-made care.
- Composed research on atomic structures and biomarkers associated with improvement.

Notwithstanding different things, these examination conditions have conveyed huge moves toward grasping the investigation of creating and making useful fixes to extend life and work major areas of strength for one. Their assessment drives the field of future science and has applications for developing related rapture.

Chapter 7

Embracing Life Expectancy Science and Craftsmanship

We want to embrace life range science and art to work on our bliss and protect the time we live on this planet. The accompanying rundown contains the primary models that help the accompanying point:

1. An exhaustive perspective Living longer and better are the two pieces of life expectancy. One's physical and profound well-being, as well as social associations and feelings of satisfaction, are considered while thinking about how long somebody will live. It is a comprehensive methodology for living a long, cheerful life.

2. Legitimate Advancement: Science plays a significant part in sorting out how to develop

functions and finding answers for deferred or decreased belongings. Research administration is fundamental in regions including food, clinical advancement, and genetic qualities to increment the future.

3. Inventive Components: For the "workmanship" of life expectancy, care, lifestyle choices, and customized well-being plans are essential. This incorporates exercises that significantly stretch and work on confidence, like pressure decrease, innovative undertakings, and empowering connections.

4. Individual Obligation: Tolerating individual obligation regarding one's well-being and achievement is a prerequisite of living a lifetime. To do this, you want to arrive at taught conclusions about your eating regimen, work-out daily schedule, and style of life. You likewise need to search for data and instruments that will assist you with living a more drawn-out, better life.

5. Social and environmental variables: Both the overall environment and society affect the future. An individual's admittance to clinical consideration, instruction, and a steady climate all influence their probability of carrying on with a more extended and better life.

6. Difficult work: Carrying on with a long life requires cautious, difficult work that adjusts craftsmanship and investigation into how to make a long life significant. Notwithstanding having a more drawn-out future, we ought to attempt to live seriously and cheerfully.

An outing is referred to as "Embracing the Science and Art of Life Expectancy" if it joins normal data with individual decisions, social help, and life expectancy science and subject matter experts. By embracing an extensive methodology to address prosperity, thriving, and individual bliss, we might attempt to live longer, better, and more joyful lives.

I. Adopting a complete strategy for maturing and wellbeing

A comprehensive technique that considers different features of physical, mental, and profound prosperity is important to living a more extended, better life. Think about the accompanying significant rules and strategies:

1. Nutrition: It is fundamental to consume a reasonable eating routine that is high in organic products, vegetables, entire grains, lean meats, and solid fats. Decrease your admission of handled food varieties, a lot of sugar, and immersed fats. Keep hydrated and contemplate advancing cell well-being through discontinuous fasting or time-confined care.

2. Exercise: Standard activity is significant for general well-being. Practices that consolidate strength, adaptability, equilibrium, and high-impact exercise are liked. To create wellness, a

propensity you can keep up with, take part in things you like.

3. Stress the board: Drawn-out pressure can exasperate various ailments. Incorporate pressure-decrease rehearses like yoga, profound breathing activities, reflection, care, and other pressure-easing exercises.

4. Focus on getting great rest. Attempt to get around 7-9 hours of solid rest every evening. Lay out an ordinary rest timetable and make your environmental elements rest well disposed of.

5. Social Associations: Maintain strong associations with loved ones. Well-being could experience the ill effects of social segregation and depression. Partake in get-togethers and lay out an organization of partners.

6. Psychological wellness: Concentrate completely on your emotional well-being. On the off chance that you need support with an

issue like nervousness or sadness, do as such. Keeping up with solid psychological wellness requires taking part in appreciation, care, and taking care of oneself.

7. Plan repetitive assessments with your medical services supplier. Your life span and personal satisfaction might be incredibly impacted by early location and the board of medical issues.

8. Preventive Consideration: Focus on preventive estimates like disease screenings, antibodies, and way-of-life changes that bring down the opportunity of persistent ailments.

9. Hydration: Hydrate over the day. For a few real cycles, water is essential.

10. Drink with some restraint and don't smoke: Both inordinate drinking and smoking are related to various medical problems. Your well-being and life span can be extraordinarily upgraded by lessening or shutting down these ways of behaving.

11. Mental Feeling: Keep your brain connected by getting new information, sorting out puzzles, or doing other mentally testing things.

Partake locally and participate in exercises that provide you with a feeling of satisfaction and motivation.

13. Positivity: Foster a hopeful point of view. Studies have demonstrated the way that confidence can work on one's well-being and life span.

Know about your environmental elements while thinking about natural variables. Consider maintainable ways of behaving and limit your openness to toxic substances and contaminations to diminish your natural effect.

15. Hereditary Variables: While qualities truly do add to life span, way of life choices can in any case hugely affect your well-being. You can

improve choices assuming you know about your family's clinical history.

16. Monetary Wellbeing: Monetary pressure can be hurtful to one's overall prosperity. To decrease monetary pressure, make arrangements for your future funds and look for help as required.

17. Side interests and Relaxation Exercises: Partake in things you need to do. Side interests and relaxation exercises are charming and stress-easing.

18. Long-lasting Learning: Keep up with your interest and learn constantly. Your whole personal satisfaction might be worked on because of keeping your cerebrum occupied.

There is no one size-fits-all methodology; remember that living a more extended, better life is a lifetime try. These rules should be modified to accommodate your specific requirements and circumstances. Customized guidance on your way to a superior, longer life can likewise be obtained by talking with medical care experts and wellbeing-trained professionals.

Ii. Probability of a change in perspective in medical care

Medical services have a colossal potential for a worldview change, which has been the subject of discussion and examination for quite a while. The probability of a significant change in the manner medical services are given, dealt with, and experienced is being energized by various patterns and conditions. Coming up next are a few significant powers and plausible focal points for a worldview change in medical care:

1. Innovation and Advanced Wellbeing: The utilization of innovation as wearables, telemedicine, electronic wellbeing records (EHRs), and wellbeing applications has previously started to change medical care. These developments empower telemedicine meetings, remote checking, and information-driven custom-made care.

2. Man-made brainpower (computer-based intelligence) and AI: Computer-based intelligence and AI commit to reforming the clinical organization, drug revelation, and the preparation of medicines. Medical care experts can go with additional exact choices as a result of man-made intelligence's quick examination of enormous datasets.

3. Genomics and Customized Medication: Genomic progressions are opening the entryway for individualized treatment. Adjusting treatments to a patient's hereditary profile can bring about additional productive and negligibly intrusive treatments.

4. Preventive and Prescient Medical services: Utilizing preventive and prescient medical services models as opposed to the more customary responsive ones can assist with distinguishing infections early and give more savvy care.

5. Patient-Driven Care: As medical care progressively takes on a patient-driven worldview, it means upgrading patient support, insight, and results. The significance of patient strengthening and shared navigation is rising.

Esteem-based care is one more procedure that intends to improve patient results while cutting costs. This change urges medical services experts to focus on well-being, preventive consideration, and productive asset designation.

7. Remote Observing and Home Consideration: Because of progressions in remote observing innovation, patients can now deal with their constant sicknesses from the comfort of their own homes. This can bring down medical services costs and clinic readmissions.

8. Interoperability and Information Sharing: Upgraded interoperability between medical services frameworks and expanded information sharing can bring about less duplication of

testing and more consistent consideration changes, as well as more educated navigation.

9. Medical services Access and Value: Endeavors to expand admittance to medical services and manage wellbeing incongruities are picking more steam. Arriving at oppressed networks is made conceivable through telemedicine, versatile facilities, and local area-based care drives.

10. Blockchain and Wellbeing Records: Blockchain innovation might work on the security and interoperability of electronic well-being records, permitting people more command over their information.

11. Emotional well-being and Comprehensive Consideration: As the worth of psychological well-being is more perceived, there is a push toward joining emotional wellness therapies with regular clinical consideration to offer more comprehensive consideration.

12. Challenges in worldwide well-being: Pandemics like the Coronavirus have underscored the requirement for stronger and adaptable medical care frameworks, pushing the advancement of telemedicine and computerized well-being arrangements.

It's essential to remember that these progressions will not happen all of a sudden, and there will be challenges and impediments to moving past, for example, legitimate limitations, protection issues, and hesitance to change. The quest for a medical care worldview change is an enticing goal for the future, due to the potential benefits concerning better quiet results, cost-productivity, and openness. Driving and accomplishing these sensational changes will rely intensely upon coordinated efforts among medical care partners, including suppliers, government officials, technologists, and patients.

B. Around What's in store

It's captivating to consider how life span will be fostered in the future as specialists keep on taking enormous steps in their insight into how the human body ages and how to extend life expectancy. While looking at the eventual fate of life span, remember the accompanying focuses:

1. Biotechnology and Hostile to Maturing Treatments: Quality treatment, regenerative medication, and prescriptions that target senescence all show huge potential for expanding human existence. To increment general well-being and life expectancy, analysts are investigating strategies to fix and recover matured cells and tissues.

2. Accuracy treatment: In the space of life span, customized treatment is acquiring significance. It is feasible to foster more powerful drugs and preventive measures by changing clinical medications and medicines as per an individual's

specific hereditary profile and well-being profile.

3. Computerized reasoning and information investigation: A gigantic measure of information about maturing and life span is being examined utilizing man-made intelligence and AI. This can be utilized to find designs, risk signs, and feasible answers for empowering solid maturing.

4. Way of life intercessions: Straightforward way of life adjustments including nourishment, exercise, and stress decrease keep on being essential in cultivating life span. There is a progressing examination into the best eating regimens and workout schedules for solid maturing.

5. Senescence Inversion: One of the primary drivers of maturing is cell senescence. Researchers are dealing with techniques to forestall or dial back senescence, which could essentially expand the solid life expectancy.

6. Life span Morals and Social Ramifications: As we increment human life span, moral quandaries and cultural issues surface. How might we guarantee that all individuals approach lifespan medicines? How might our medical services and retirement frameworks be changed to oblige expanded life expectancies? Resolving these problems will be fundamental.

7. support for Maturing Exploration: As the advantages of maturing research become all the more clear, both public and confidential help for it is expected to rise. Logical progressions connected with maturing can be accelerated by subsidizing.

8. Networks and Associations Zeroed in on Life span: Networks and associations with a life span center are shaping, and uniting scientists, money managers, and fans to participate in and advance life span research.

9. Worldwide Collaboration: Life span is a worldwide issue, so global participation is vital.

To build our insight into maturing and give productive arrangements, analysts and policymakers from everywhere in the world are teaming up.

10. Mind-Body Association: It's urgent to comprehend how life span and psychological well-being are connected. Future headways in life expectancy will vigorously rely upon strategies for improving mental and psychological well-being.

While there have been significant advances in the investigation of life span, it is pivotal to recall that there is still a lot to learn and that the work to increase the human lifetime is muddled and varied. The eventual fate of life span will likewise be extraordinarily affected by moral issues, lawful limitations, and popular assessment.

Life span research can change how we view maturing, how we approach medical care, and how we view the human experience. Planning for a lifespan is eventually a confident endeavor.

I. Hold back nothing in the investigation of life expectancy

As they can change medical services, upgrade personal satisfaction, and address the issues welcomed by a maturing populace, progressions in life span research are of gigantic interest. We should discuss a few expected improvements in lifespan research because of the latest things and dynamic examination nearby. If it's not too much trouble, remember that logical exploration is a powerful field and that there might have been significant headways past this.

1. Accuracy Medication: Genomic and customized medication improvements are expected to be influential for the field of life span research. Customized medications and medicines are currently potential because of the developing utilization of hereditary data by researchers to pinpoint specific reasons for extraordinary maturing processes.

2. Senescence and Cell Maturing: Researchers are inspecting cell senescence, the interaction through which cells bit by bit lose their ability to multiply and proceed as expected. Senolytic treatments, which target senescent cells, might be viable in broadening solid life.

3. Research on telomeres: Telomeres are defensive covers on the finishes of chromosomes that get more limited as cells partition. Maturing and telomere shortening are connected. Scientists are investigating ways of halting or stopping telomere shortening, which could build the life span of cells and other living things.

4. Calorie Limitation and Diet: Research on calorie limitation and irregular fasting proposes they might have life span expansion benefits. Mimetics, or substances that repeat the impacts of caloric limitation, are being created by analysts as imminent treatments while they explore the sub-atomic components hidden in these impacts.

5. Regenerative Medication: Improvements in undeveloped cell and tissue designing are setting out new open doors for the recovery of hurt or maturing tissues and organs. Healthspan (the piece of life during which one is typically sound), as well as life expectancy, may both be expanded subsequently.

6. Senescence Pathways and Therapeutics: The instruments and pathways that add to maturing are as yet being contemplated. The formation of meds that lull or converse the maturing system might result from the recognizable proof of explicit focuses inside these pathways.

7. Man-made consciousness and AI: Man-made intelligence and ML are used to inspect enormous datasets relating to maturing and life span. By utilizing these apparatuses, patterns and potential mediations that traditional examination strategies could have missed can be found.

8. Biotechnology and nanotechnology are investigating how to make state-of-the-art cures, for example, nanobots that can fix cells and tissues at the sub-atomic level or convey prescriptions precisely to the piece of the body where fundamental.

9. Social and natural impacts: Scientists are likewise looking at how an individual's way of

life, social conditions, and climate influence their capacity to carry on with a long life. More noteworthy exhaustive ways of expanding solid life expectancy might result from information on these issues.

10. Moral and Social Contemplations: As life span research propels, moral and social worries concerning how to scatter and make these advancements accessible to the public will turn out to be more critical. The discussion will zero in vigorously on guaranteeing fair access and managing possible results.

The expansion of human lifetime far past existing standards remains a difficult undertaking with different moral, functional, and logical ramifications, notwithstanding the way that there have been significant advances in this field. Future advances in this space will likely require interdisciplinary collaboration and further examination into the mind-boggling science of maturing.

Ii. The general public's devotion to advancing a culture of long life

Society assumes a basic part in advancing a culture of long life by molding the circumstances, outlooks, and standards of conduct that influence individuals' prosperity and success as they age. Overall people who energize and love driving a long, solid, and productive life are alluded to as having a culture of life span. Coming up next are a few indispensable ways that society ought to help this culture:

1. Advancing Sound Lifestyles: Advancing sound lifestyles should be possible in the public eye through broad well-being drives, instructive drives, and decisions that help work out a solid eating regimen, and stress decrease. It's likewise critical to search out nutritious feasts, painstakingly thought to be clinical considerations and safe sporting facilities.

2. Killing ageism: Ageism, or bias against individuals in light of their age, can be negative to the individual satisfaction of additional carefully prepared individuals. Society can neutralize ageism by reinforcing intergenerational compassion and strength, advancing sweeping circumstances, and wiping out winning developing biases.

3. Creating Profound dependability: Profound prosperity is an essential part of life expectancy. Associations and organizations can give mental

prosperity administrations, reduce the shame related with close-to-home prosperity issues, and cultivate opportunities for social collaboration and regular consolation.

4. Medical care administration Access: Ensuring that everybody approaches suitable clinical consideration is fundamental for broadening life. Individuals can keep up with their well-being as they age with the assistance of sensible drugs, broad clinical consideration drives, and routine clinical assessments.

5. Advancing Profound Learning: Improvement and profound learning are significant for emotional well-being and can expand an individual's dynamic and useful years. Society can uphold this by allowing individuals of any age the opportunity to foster their abilities and master new things.

6. Social Affiliation: Social disconnection and sadness can hurt an individual's physical and general success. Improvement of causal

associations and neighborhood local area advancement are urged to address these worries. Programs that pair seniors with those of practically identical age and more youthful ages can be particularly helpful.

7. Workforce Plans: If individuals so decide, arrangements that help more seasoned laborers, including adaptable retirement choices, age-accommodating work environments, and opportunities for proficient headway, may urge them to keep turning out gainfully for longer.

8. Metropolitan preparation: Creating age-accommodating networks with open travel, safe streets, and nearby conveniences can work on the individual joy of older residents and urge them to keep a functioning and connected lifestyle.

9. Monetary Soundness: A vital calculation deciding life expectancy is monetary dependability. Seniors' monetary security can be expanded through friendly well-being nets,

retirement hold finances projects, and lodging choices.

10. Development and Progress: Embracing development and progress can assist with addressing issues connecting with the new period, for example, telemedicine, wearable wellbeing innovation, and savvy home advancement.

11. Intergenerational Affiliations: Encouraging ties between various age gatherings can support understanding and supporting each other. Programs that bring youthful and elderly folks together for cooperation, coaching, and preparation may be exceptionally valuable.

The progression of a culture of long life can be significantly helped by society by advancing sound living, resolving age-related issues, and regarding the achievements of more established residents. A culture of life expectancy helps more prepared grown-ups as well as society in general by drawing on the information and experience of its developing populace and propelling the success of all of its residents.

Iii. Propelling individuals to assume responsibility for their prosperity and life expectancy

It is fundamental to advance general prosperity and forestall persistent illnesses that individuals are spurred to assume responsibility for their well-being and life span. To urge individuals to roll out sure improvements in their lives, think about the accompanying strategies and exhortation:

1. Instruction and Mindfulness: Start by expanding public comprehension of the worth of well-being and life span. Illuminate others on the

benefits of a solid way of life, the risks of destructive things to do, and the impact of qualities on life expectancy. Utilize different stages to spread this data, including local area occasions, studios, courses, and online entertainment.

Assist with putting forth reasonable objectives for their well-being and life expectancy by encouraging them on the most proficient method to do so. Urge them to start little with unmistakable, quantifiable, and possible objectives. Frequently, slow progression is more persevering than sudden change.

3. Nutrition: Support a decent eating routine brimming with new leafy foods, lean meats, entire grains, and great fats. Advance smart eating, reasonable partitioning, and the benefit of remaining hydrated. give enlightening materials like healthy recipe guides and counsel on food arranging.

4. Active work: Advance continuous active work. Whether it's moving, swimming, yoga, or some other movement, urge people to find something they appreciate doing. Urge them to remember to practice for their ordinary schedules and accentuate the worth of consistency.

5. Stress The board: Present practices for lessening pressure, like care, profound breathing, and moderate muscle unwinding. Tending to pressure is fundamental since it can unfavorably affect well-being and life span.

6. Customary Check-ups: Urge individuals to make arrangements for normal check-ups with clinically trained professionals. Early conclusions of medical conditions and routine tests can incredibly improve results. Illuminate the general population on the importance of immunizations, malignant growth screenings, and age-proper well-being assessments.

Stress the significance of appropriate rest
cleanliness in point seven. Support keeping a
customary rest plan, making a comfortable
dozing space, and scaling back screen time
before bed. Different medical problems can
result from unfortunate rest.

8. Social Associations: Accentuate how
significant social ties are to life span. Urge them
to keep solid ties with their loved ones. Physical
and profound well-being can be adversely
affected by friendly segregation and dejection.

9. Keep away from Negative Propensities:
Advise them regarding the risks of smoking,
exorbitant liquor utilization, and illicit drug use.
Give individuals who need to shut down these
perilous ways of behaving help and assets.

10. Psychological well-being: Increment public
attention to psychological wellness concerns and
diminish disgrace related to getting treatment for
them. Standard emotional wellness registrations

are empowered, and benefits are made accessible.

11. Monetary Preparation: Discuss the monetary features of well-being and life span, like the meaning of putting something aside for retirement clinical costs. Admittance to medical services and general prosperity can be influenced by monetary soundness.

12. Local area Backing: Lay out an organization or local area that is empowering so that individuals might discuss their encounters, wins, and hardships as they seek long-haul well-being. Peer backing might be unbelievably motivating.

13. Set the Bar High: Set the bar high by carrying on with a sound way of life yourself. To propel and draw in individuals, discuss your achievements and battles.

Perceive that everybody's way to well-being and life span is unique and adopt a customized strategy. Change direction and help to every individual's special requirements and circumstances.

15. Observe Achievement: Commend any achievements or achievements you might have along the course. Inspiration and confidence can be expanded by uplifting feedback.

It takes a multi-layered procedure that addresses physical, mental, and social prosperity to empower individuals to assume responsibility for their well-being and life expectancy. Individuals' lives can change essentially while close to nothing, enduring changes are supported and ceaseless help is advertised.

V. The worth of collective endeavors in developing an additional prosperous and expanded future

Numerous variables contribute essentially to the embellishment of a more extended and better future. The accompanying urgent subtleties underline their importance:

Complex Issues Call for Cooperative Arrangements: Current overall emergencies in general well-being, destitution, and environmental change are only a couple of the dire issues that mankind is managing. People or detached associations alone can't effectively tackle these issues. To resolve these mind-boggling issues, aggregate endeavors unite different perspectives, resources, and abilities.

2. Asset Pooling: Bunch drives consider the consolidating of both monetary and scholarly

assets. Thus, greater ventures are conceivable and can have a greater effect. Assets from associations, organizations, states, and people can be in every way pooled to subsidize drives and exploration that might have a drawn-out result.

3. Information Trade: The trade of data and information is worked with by joint effort. As different associations and individuals consolidate, they each contribute their specific information and viewpoints. Inventive arrangements and a more prominent understanding of mind-boggling issues are much of the time created because of this thought of cross-fertilization.

4. Synergy: At the point when individuals cooperate, they can collaborate, which is what is going on in which the general aftereffect of their endeavors is higher than the completion of their singular ones. By cooperating, you can create collaborations, efficiencies, and results that working alone wouldn't have the option to.

5. Social cohesiveness: Teaming up to accomplish shared goals advances a feeling of social cohesiveness and fortitude. To make a superior future, it can upgrade connections to the local area, trust, and a sensation of direction.

6. Aggregate activities can affect foundational changes and administrative changes. Various gatherings that meet up on the side of a common objective can come down to legislatures and organizations to institute changes and strategies that advance long-haul supportability, value, and prosperity.

7. extended Term Vision: Aggregate activities regularly incorporate preparation and venture over an extended timeframe. They are bound to focus on supportability and consider the necessities of people in the future when different partners consent to a bound-together vision.

8. Resilience: Even with unanticipated challenges, flexibility can be worked on through

cooperative endeavors. When confronted with moving circumstances and new difficulties, a fluctuated organization of donors is better ready to adjust and manage them.

9. Worldwide Difficulties Need Worldwide Arrangements: A considerable lot of the most serious issues the world contends, similar to pandemics and environmental change, are worldwide in scope. Purposeful endeavors should be made on an overall scale to resolve these issues, which calls for worldwide participation.

10. Interconnectedness: In the present universally interconnected globe, a solitary association or country's activities can have broad impacts. The need to gather activities to make a reasonable and fruitful future for everybody is featured in the acknowledgment of this reliance.

It is difficult to misrepresent how vital gathering exercises are to making an additional prosperous and expanded future. Tending to complex worldwide difficulties, cultivating strength, and pursuing a more manageable and only world for people in the future all rely upon joint effort, participation, and aggregate activity.

The End